THE TRUTH ABOUT VASECTOMY

THE
TRUTH
ABOUT
VASECTOMY

Louis J. Rosenfeld, M.D., F.A.C.S.
and
Marvin Grosswirth

Prentice-Hall, Inc.
Englewood Cliffs, N.J.

The Truth About Vasectomy by Louis J. Rosenfeld, M.D.
and Marvin Grosswirth

Copyright © 1972 by Louis J. Rosenfeld, M.D.
and Marvin Grosswirth

Printed in the United States of America

Prentice-Hall International, Inc., London
Prentice-Hall of Australia, Pty. Ltd., North Sydney
Prentice-Hall of Canada, Ltd., Toronto
Prentice-Hall of India Private Ltd., New Delhi
Prentice-Hall of Japan, Inc., Tokyo

Library of Congress Cataloging in Publication Data

Rosenfeld, Louis J.,
    The truth about vasectomy.

    Includes bibliographies.
    1. Vasectomy. I. Grosswirth, Marvin,
joint author. II. Title. [DNLM: 1. Sterilization,
Sexual—Popular works. 2. Vas deferens—Surgery—
Popular works. WJ 780 R 813t 1972]
RD571.R68   613.9'42   72-8341
ISBN 0-13-931170-X

To
Elizabeth Rosenfeld
who pushed
and
Marilyn Grosswirth
who pulled

AUTHORS' NOTE

Every effort has been made to produce a book that is interesting and informative for the average layman. We believe that this cannot be accomplished if the reader is constantly required to interrupt his train of thought by checking explanatory footnotes or glossaries. Therefore, whenever a word or phrase that we think needs explaining occurs, the explanation appears in the text, immediately following the term. If the term is used again far enough along so that the reader may have forgotten its meaning, the definition is repeated.

Footnotes that appear throughout the book refer only to original source material. The reader need not concern himself with them unless he wishes to read further on the particular subject under discussion, in which case the footnotes will provide an excellent bibliography.

We are indebted to many people for their assistance in the research and preparation of this book. The Association for Voluntary Sterilization (AVS) exhibited patience and understanding far beyond the call of duty. Among the individuals who lent their unique talents to this work are (alphabetically):

Elizabeth Barrett, medical researcher, who supplied us

7

with so much information that we finally had to ask her to stop so that we could get on with the book; Jim Bouton; Mrs. Evelyn Bryant, MSW, a social worker for AVS; Helen Edey, M.D., chairman of AVS's Executive Committee; Matthew Freund, Ph.D., Professor of Pharmacology, Associate Professor of Obstetrics and Gynecology, New York Medical College; Bernard Fruchtman, M.D., who encouraged and abetted us and who read the first draft; Donald H. Higgins, Public Relations Director, AVS, who supplied enough material to halve the time we would have had to spend on research and who patiently answered innumerable questions; John R. Rague, Executive Director of AVS; Howard Rowe, Ph.D., director of Genetic Laboratories, Inc.; Robert M. Siegmann, who read the manuscript and offered many helpful suggestions and comments; Jerome K. Silbert, M.D., director of laboratories for Idant Corp.; Mrs. Jeanne Swinton, librarian of the Margaret Sanger Research Bureau, New York, who opened her voluminous files to us and directed us toward other sources of material; and Herbert N. Weber, M.D., who shared some of his professional experiences with us.

Although we cannot name them, we are deeply grateful to the many friends, colleagues and patients who shared their views and experiences with us.

Marilyn Grosswirth was instrumental in getting our sentences properly structured, in having words like *anesthesia* spelled correctly, and in making sure that points obvious to us were equally clear to the reader.

All of these people made this book possible. But we assume full responsibility for any errors in information or in judgment which may have crept in.

Louis J. Rosenfeld, M.D.
Marvin Grosswirth

New York

All names of individual patients
mentioned in the case histories have
been changed to protect their privacy

TABLE OF CONTENTS

I

SOME QUESTIONS AND ANSWERS

Here are some often-asked questions about vasectomies —and their answers. Almost all of the questions are answered more fully in the following chapters. The number in parentheses after an answer indicates the chapter in which more information will be found.

1. What is a vasectomy?
It is a simple surgical procedure that makes a man sterile. (4)

2. How is it done?
A surgeon severs and ties off two narrow tubes located in the scrotum, preventing the passage of sperm. (4)

3. Why would anyone want such an operation?
To insure against unwanted pregnancies when other methods of birth control are unusable and uncertain. (2)

4. But aren't researchers working on a male contraceptive pill?

13

Yes. But there are three factors to consider: First, we do not know how expensive such a pill will be. Second, there is no way of knowing any given individual's reaction to, or tolerance of, such a pill. Third, and most important, there is no way of predicting when such a pill will be on the market. While you're waiting for it, you could become a father. (2)

5. But sterilization—that's like castration, isn't it?
Absolutely not. There is no connection between sterilization and castration. The testicles, which produce the male hormones, are not affected in any way. (3, 4)

6. Do you mean to say there's no connection between fertility and masculinity?
Physiologically, no; psychologically, however, it depends on you. If you think there is a connection, then there is. If you have confidence in your own masculinity, then the vasectomy will not affect it —except, possibly, for the better. But that, too, is psychological. (3, 4, 6, 8, 10)

7. What will my wife think of me if I become sterile?
That depends upon your wife, upon you, and upon your relationship together. A woman who is concerned about unwanted pregnancies usually responds very well to her husbands' vasectomy. (7, 8, 10)

8. But won't she be put off by my deformity?
There is no deformity. The surgeon makes two tiny incisions in the scrotum. When those incisions heal—in a matter of days—there is no way anyone will know that a vasectomy has been performed ex-

cept by being told or by closely inspecting the scrotum with a magnifying glass for the tiny scars that may remain.

9. Will a vasectomy affect my sex life?
In most cases, no. In many cases, however, vasectomy has a very positive affect on sexual activity. Relations are more frequent and more enjoyable for both partners. (6, 7, 8)

10. What effect will a vasectomy have on my sexual performance?
Physiologically, none. Psychologically, it could have a tremendous affect. Many vasectomized men claim that they are more virile, more interested in sex, have larger, firmer erections, take longer to reach orgasm, and have orgasms that last longer. On occasion, a man with a sexual problem will become impotent after a vasectomy. But that's because of his mind, not his body. (6, 9, 10)

11. How long would I have to be hospitalized?
Probably not at all. The vast majority of vasectomies are performed in the doctor's office and take about twenty minutes. (4)

12. Does it hurt much?
It doesn't hurt at all. The doctor will administer a local anesthetic, which will eliminate all pain in the area of the surgery while allowing you to be fully awake during the procedure. (4)

13. Once the local anesthetic wears off, is there any pain?
A little, and for a short time. A mild analgesic, such as two aspirin tablets, will relieve the pain in most cases. (4)

14. You say the operation is simple—but is it safe?
Some 3 percent of all vasectomized men have some
after-effects—swelling, low-grade infection, a little
bleeding of the incision. Almost none of these rare
aftereffects is serious. (4)

15. How soon can I resume my normal functions?
As long as you do nothing too strenuous, you can
go back to work the next day. Most men have their
vasectomies on Friday afternoons. They relax over
the weekend, and by Monday morning they're
ready for action. (4)

16. Does that include sex?
Yes. It's best to wait until the incisions heal, but
that only takes a day or two for most men. Some
doctors recommend waiting from five to seven days
after healing before resuming sexual activity. (4)

*17. And then my worries about unwanted pregnancy
are over, right?*
Wrong. There is a sizable quantity of sperm stored
in your sex organs past the point of the vasectomy.
You'll have to use contraceptives until your doctor
gives you a negative sperm count. *Then* your worries are over. (4)

18. Is a dry orgasm as good as a normal one?
We don't know, but the question is academic.
Vasectomized men ejaculate just as they did prior
to the operation. (4, 6, 8)

19. But if there's no more sperm coming out . . . ?
Sperm makes up only a small portion of the total
ejaculate, so that neither you nor your partner will
be able to discern any difference in the quantity of
ejaculate. (3, 4)

20. What happens to the sperm?
Sperm cells are reabsorbed by the body into the bloodstream and passed out with body waste, exactly the same as all the other cells in your body that are being constantly renewed and replaced. (3, 4)

21. If I change my mind later, can I have the vasectomy reversed?
You can try, and it may be successful, but the odds are heavily against it. Men who have vasectomies should consider the procedure as permanent and irreversible. (9)

22. But I read that there are valves and plugs that accomplish the same results as vasectomies but are removable if you change your mind.
These are all in the experimental stage and none has yet been proven. They are not available to the general public and no one is prepared to predict when they will be. (9)

23. Couldn't my wife be sterilized instead of me?
Yes. A recently developed technique makes female sterilization nearly as fast and as easy as vasectomy. But this method is not available except in a few widely scattered clinics. In the next year or two, it will probably be as easy for a woman to become sterilized as it now is for a man. In the meantime, female sterilization usually takes longer and costs more. (2, 4)

24. How much does a vasectomy cost?
Anywhere from $50 to $250, depending upon where you have it done. Some clinics will perform vasectomies free for those who cannot afford to pay.

25. Two hundred and fifty dollars—isn't that kind of expensive?
That depends upon what you compare it with. Certainly the average married couple spends at least that on contraceptives during their sexually active years. Compared to the cost of an unplanned child, the price of a vasectomy is infinitesimal. And the cost of fear and anxiety over an unwanted pregnancy cannot be measured in dollars and cents. (7, 8)

26. How many men have been vasectomized?
According to the Association for Voluntary Sterilization, by 1969, two to three million people have been sterilized, most of whom were men. In 1970 750,000 men had vasectomies, followed by another 800,000 in 1971. AVS projects a million more vasectomies for 1972. And these figures are just for the United States. Millions of men have been and are being vasectomized in countries throughout the world.

27. I take it, then, that vasectomies are legal?
Vasectomies are legal in all fifty states. (5)

28. Do I have to sign anything?
All surgery requires that a release be signed. For a vasectomy, most physicians and clinics will ask you and your wife to sign a release. A typical vasectomy release form is shown in Appendix A.

29. Is a vasectomy ever performed in connection with other surgery?
Frequently. The most common incidence is in conjunction with a prostatectomy. (3)
   If you expect to be operated on for an inguinal hernia, the surgeon can probably perform a vasec-

tomy at the same time, but only if you ask him to do so.

30. Can any doctor perform a vasectomy?
Any *surgeon* can, but it is advisable to seek out a urologist, one who has had some experience with vasectomies. (4, 5)

31. I don't know any urologists. How can I find one?
Ask your family physician to recommend one. If he can't or won't, check with your local county or state medical society. If you still can't find one, contact the nearest office of Planned Parenthood, Zero Population Growth, or any other birth control agency. If there are none near you, write to the Association for Voluntary Sterilization, Inc., 14 W. 40th St. New York, N.Y. 10018; telephone (212) 524-2344.

   If you prefer a clinic or hospital, check the list in Appendix B.

32. What do you mean, "can't or won't"? Are there doctors who are against vasectomies?
Roman Catholics, Orthodox Jews, and practicing Muslims are opposed to all forms of birth control—for religious reasons, not for medical ones. (5)

33. What about single men—can they get vasectomies?
Yes, but with difficulty. Many doctors have established arbitrary standards—in addition to marital status—of age, family size, income, etc., to determine whether they will perform a particular vasectomy.

34. Will my health insurance cover a vasectomy?
Probably. Most health insurance programs will pay

for at least part of the cost. So will Medicare and Medicaid, but circumstances vary from state to state. Check with your insurance company and your local Medicare/Medicaid offices to determine the extent of their coverage.

35. What long-lasting effects can I expect if I have a vasectomy?

If you are like most men who have been vasectomized, you will be totally free of any concern about unwanted pregnancies. You can expect an improvement in your sex life, in your wife's sexual responsiveness, and in your general sense of well-being.

And you may derive some small satisfaction from the knowledge that you are making a valuable contribution to the human race, which at this very moment, as you read this, is in danger of breeding itself off the face of the earth.

2

A BRIEF HISTORY OF CONTRACEPTION

The terms "birth control" and "contraception" are often used interchangeably, frequently with considerable inaccuracy. "Birth control" is exactly what the two words suggest: the control of birth. A more sophisticated definition would be control of the birth *rate*. Thus, anything from sexual abstention to infanticide qualifies as a method of birth control.

Contraception—literally, "against conception"—is only one method of birth control. Unquestionably, Western culture regards contraception as the most favored method, from every point of view—ethical, aesthetic, moral, and religious. Even the most enthusiastic supporters of legalized abortion agree that it is better for all concerned not to have conceived in the first place. And while the opponents of abortion— those who regard it as nothing but another version of infanticide—are not necessarily in favor of contraception, they are nevertheless considerably less vehement in their opposition to it. If the church can be regarded as a reflection of society as a whole, then it is significant that only the most orthodox segments of organized religion are opposed to contraception, whereas those who oppose abortion represent a cross-section of every shade of religious persuasion.

Infanticide, the willful and deliberate destruction of new-born babies, is completely out of the question. No one even mentions it, although it was certainly a part of our history. Every schoolboy knows the tales of the ancient Spartans, who left unwanted infants on hillsides, to perish from exposure. Aristotle "was forced to recommend . . . the death of unwanted babies through exposure—a practice common even today among many primitive tribes." [1]* But the abortion of the fetus or the prevention of conception has always been more acceptable. The long, complex history of birth control (which we can only survey here) is a chronology of man's efforts to inhibit birth without inhibiting sex.

No one knows exactly when man first associated the ejaculation of the male's semen with the birth of a baby. (Many people use the words *sperm* and *semen* interchangeably, but they are not the same. Sperm, which is short for *spermatozoon,* is a cell that fertilizes the egg in the female's body, thus causing conception. Semen is the fluid that carries the sperm. Both are discussed in greater detail in the next chapter. For now, it is enough to understand the difference and to realize that there are millions of sperm in a single ejaculation and that it takes only one to make a woman pregnant.) Even today, some primitive societies have no idea that sexual intercourse results in childbirth. It is not surprising: nine months is a long time over which to connect the two events.

It would have been reasonable for our early ancestors to assume that infants were somehow self-generated within the mother's womb, that strange mechanism which bleeds with the cycles of the moon, which causes the abdomen to swell,

---

* References appear at the end of the chapter.

and which finally, after much pain and discomfort, issues forth a child. Obviously, some sort of magic had to be involved in childbirth, and just as obviously, only magic could prevent its recurrence. Charms, amulets, potions, and rituals were evolved, some of which persisted, with variations, through the Middle Ages.

If the magic was imprecise, its purpose was not: man has wanted to limit the size of his family since recorded time and very likely before, because the earliest examples of the written word include contraceptive techniques and practices.

It is also clear that by the time writing had been invented there was no doubt that semen and conception were connected. An Egyptian papyrus written about 1850 B.C. contains several prescriptions and recipes for contraceptives. The medications described are intended for placement in the vagina—a clear indication that the ancient physicians knew about the fertilizing quality of semen (although exactly how it functioned, as well as the existence of sperm, remained a mystery until the invention of the microscope). Among the potions offered were concoctions consisting of crocodile dung, and a variety of oils and honey.

Whether by accident or by design, the ancients actually hit upon several partially effective techniques. For one thing, they advised that the potions be poured over a *pessary,* or plug, to be inserted in the vagina. The plugging action by itself would have some limited contraceptive value. Oily, sticky substances inhibit the smooth flow of sperm in the vaginal canal. The acid in crocodile dung is a mild spermicide, although the substance itself must have caused numerous infections.

Another papyrus, written in 1550 B.C. and discovered at Luxor, Egypt, in 1873, advised the use of a recipe based on "tips of acacia." The acacia is a shrub that "when fermented and dissolved in water, liberates lactic acid, a substance frequently used in early twentieth-century spermicides." [2] However, the ancient Egyptians also used many amulets and charms. There is no way of knowing whether the Egyptians' partially effective contraceptive techniques were based on more or less scientific study, or were merely near-direct hits by a few of the many arrows let loose by the early physicians, most of which fell wide of the mark.

Once it was established that semen and childbirth were related, it required no particular genius to realize that *coitus interruptus*—withdrawing the penis from the vagina immediately prior to orgasm—would prevent conception. One of the earliest records of this method of birth control appears in the Bible (Genesis 38:8–10): And Judah said unto Onan, Go in unto thy brother's wife, and marry her, and raise up seed to thy brother. And Onan knew that the seed should not be his; and it came to pass when he went in unto his brother's wife, that he spilled it on the ground, lest that he should give seed to his brother. And the thing which he did displeased the Lord: wherefore he slew him also.

The so-called "sin" of Onan has stirred considerable controversy, most of which is little known today. Modern interpretations of this passage see it as a clear injunction against contraception and masturbation (often referred to as onanism), but this view is relatively recent. Initially, Onan's sin was his refusal to accept the principle of *levirate*, "the sometimes compulsory marriage of a widow by the brother of her deceased husband." [3] This practice, common among ancient peoples, enabled a widow to continue to remain part of her late husband's family and provided for her care. "Later some Rabbis laid stress on the act of coitus interruptus, especially where it was medically indicated." [4] "Certain writers in the Talmud forbade intra-vaginal ejaculation during the first twenty-four months that a woman nursed her child, and advised the husband to 'thresh inside but winnow outside.' " [5]

Coitus interruptus continued to be practiced throughout history in all parts of the world, and is still one of the most popular contraceptive techniques in use, even among fairly well-educated societies where more sophisticated techniques are available. There are problems affecting the efficacy of coitus interruptus; according to many experts, the psychological aspects are among the least of them. Many couples have apparently adjusted quite happily to the man having his orgasm a good distance away from his partner's vagina.

The problems are primarily physiological. First, it takes superb timing to be able to withdraw at *precisely* the moment of orgasm. A millisecond too late can mean trouble, because most sperm cells are ejaculated at the beginning of the orgasm. Furthermore, the penis emits a preorgasmic fluid that acts as a lubricant but can carry some sperm. If any of the semen comes into contact with the vulva, even on the outside, fertilization can occur. Those sperm are persistent, with but a single purpose for their existence. So, while coitus interruptus is not without some value as a contraceptive method, it has considerably less than a 100 percent success rate, as many would-be Onans who are now fathers can testify.

Prescriptions taken internally were also popular in Talmudic times, particularly because they helped to solve the controversy surrounding birth control. It was considered the man's duty to propagate the race. No such responsibility burdened the woman, however—not because women were considered special, but because they were considered incapable of bearing responsibility. Therefore, if a man were to have intercourse with his wife in the accepted manner, he would have fulfilled his religious and patriotic obligations. If, however, his wife had taken some contraceptive measure, it was not his fault. Nor could she be punished, because she did not have the responsibility in the first place. The so-called "cup of roots," a concoction of herbs, became a popular drink among the Hebrew women of antiquity.

An often-told story is that of Rabbi Hiyya and Judith, his wife (circa 200 A.D.). After a rather difficult childbirth, Judith appeared before her husband in disguise and asked: "Are women included in the commandment of propagation?" "They are not," replied the sage. Judith went home, took the cup of roots, and allegedly became sterile. The good rabbi's only recorded comment was: "I wish you had allowed me one more birth."

Rabbi Yohanan, an accomplished physician who lived in the third century, prescribed a concoction of Alexandrian gum of the *Spina Aegypta,* liquid alum, and garden crocus. The mixture, taken with three cups of wine, was claimed to be a curative for gonorrhea. Taken with two cups of beer, it was supposed not only to cure jaundice but to induce sterility. There are no records as to the efficacy of this medication.

Many of these contraceptive methods—coitus interruptus, plugs, pessaries, ointments and oils, potions and medicines— were widely used by the Greeks and Romans. Somewhat more exotic prescriptions continued to appear, however. Pliny the Elder (23–79 A.D.) offered the following:

> From a spider called Phalangium, described as having a hairy body and an enormous head, are to be extracted two small worms. These, attached to a piece of deer's skin, before sunrise, to a woman's body, will prevent conception.[6]

No doubt . . . but we suspect that contraception in this case resulted from abstinence. Given a choice between an unwanted pregnancy and having to wear two worms taken from a hairy, large-headed spider, most women probably opted for a cold shower.

Among the most influential of the ancients in matters of contraception was Pandarios Dioscorides, a Greek pharmacologist of the first century A.D. whose "Greek Herbal" was in use throughout Europe and the Muslim world until the sixteenth century. Soranos of Ephesus (98–138 A.D.), a Roman physician during the reigns of Trajan and Hadrian, has been described as "the greatest gynecologist of antiquity." Many of his prescriptions were of dubious value, but his basic principles were sound, based on blockage of the vaginal canal and on the use of various astringents to reduce the size of the cervical opening.

Even sheaths were known to the ancient Romans. The reader is most likely to associate the word "sheath" with the condom, a male contraceptive device that will be discussed in detail shortly. But as late as the nineteenth century, women were inserting sheaths in their vaginas to catch the semen and prevent its entry into the uterus.

In the second century, Antoninus Liberalis (better known as Ovid) wrote his *Metamorphoses,* which includes the story of Pasiphaë and Minos, the king of Crete, whose semen was supposed to contain snakes and spiders. Instead of fathering children, as every good king should, he left a trail of severely injured women. Finally, someone decided to try an experiment. A goat's bladder was inserted into a woman's vagina and it proved an adequate receptacle to contain the king's semen. He promptly sought out his wife Pasiphaë, daughter of the king of the sun. While she had been immune to the effects of Minos's unpleasant emissions, their marriage had nevertheless been fruitless. The goat's bladder was promptly popped into place and the happy couple eventually had eight children. Apparently the membrane was strong enough to retain the snakes and spiders, but not the intrepid little sperm. Difficult as this story may be to accept, it nevertheless clearly demonstrates that the use of a sheath, made of animal membrane, was known.

From about the time of the birth of Christ until the invention of the condom in the sixteenth century, contraceptive methods were largely the same in every culture and civilization. Among the scores, perhaps hundreds, of medications prescribed, some came remarkably close to the mark. Aetios of Amida, a sixth-century Byzantine physician, prescribed vinegar and brine as a precoital douche. Both substances are highly spermicidal and probably would have been more popular had they not caused some burning sensations on the sensitive membranes of the genitals.

Chinese, Indian, and Muslim writers tended to duplicate each other, and all of them, even the great ones, included some incredible nonsense with otherwise sound advice. For example, many writers believed that a woman who remained passive during intercourse would refrain from agitating the semen, thereby discouraging its entrance into the uterus. Still others believed that vigorous movement during intercourse would cause the semen to be expelled. Jumping up and down, induced sneezing, and various postures and positions were all recommended. Ibn al-Jami, an otherwise brilliant Jewish-Egyptian physician in the court of Saladin (1171–1193), wrote that beans eaten on an empty stomach would cause female sterility. (Once again, the authors must conclude that the ultimate contraceptive method here was abstinence. Beans eaten on an empty stomach are likely to produce results, other than sterility, which would make a woman something less than desirable.)

In 1564, credit for the invention of the condom was given to Gabriello Fallopio (1523–1562), an Italian anatomist whose other claim to fame was the discovery of the Fallopian tubes, the two little ducts that connect the uterus to the ovaries. His book was published two years after his death. Its title, *De Morbo Gallico Liber Absolutismus,* freely translates to: "The Complete Book of Syphilis." (Syphilis was known as the French, or Gallic, disease all over Europe—except in France, where it was called the English disease.) In this book, Fallopio describes a sheath made of linen and cut to fit the shape of the *glans* (the head of the penis). He claimed to have invented the device as a prevention against syphilis, and asserted that none of the 1100 men who tried it became infected.

The word "condom" remains something of an etymological mystery. It is believed to come from the name of one Dr. Condon (or Conton or Condom) who is said to have developed sheaths from animal membrane, but there is little evidence to support the accuracy of this story. In any case, regardless of who invented it or named it, both the invention and the name grew rapidly in popularity and in use. By the middle of the eighteenth century, English wits were praising and ridiculing the condom in songs and poems. Condom shops proliferated all over London and in other major cities of Europe, and by 1770 some were advertising their wares publicly.

A dictionary of slang, published in 1811, carries the following entry:

> CUNDUM. The dried gut of a sheep, worn by men in the act of coition, to prevent venereal disease . . . These machines were long prepared and sold by a matron of the name of Philips, at the Green Canister, in Half-moon-Street, in the Strand. That

good lady having acquired a fortune, retired from
business; but learning that the town was not well
served by her successors, she, out of a patriotic zeal
for the public welfare, returned to her occupation;
of which she gave notice by divers hand-bills, in
circulation in the year 1776.[7]

History does not record when or by whom the condom
was first perceived as a contraceptive, but it was widely used
as such shortly after its appearance on the market. Casanova
(1725–1798) used them and praised them in his writings. He
knew about other methods of contraception as well, including block pessaries and cervical caps, which he improvised
by squeezing the juice from half a lemon and inserting the
caplike rind in the vagina.

In 1843–1844, Goodyear and Hancock developed the vul-
canization of rubber and, doubtless without realizing it, revo-
lutionized birth control. Condoms could now be manufactured cheaply, efficiently, and in large quantities. Other
rubber devices, notably the diaphragm and cervical cap, were
also developed through a long series of experiments and
through trial and error. While modern technology has rendered these products near-perfect, there is still some risk
attached to their use. Condoms have been known to leak,
through holes so tiny as to be invisible to the naked eye.
(Sperm, remember, are microscopic.) Sometimes condoms
slip off immediately after intercourse when the penis is
removed from the vagina; the slightest drop of spillage can
cause pregnancy. Men have also been known, in the heat of
the moment, to forget to apply the condom.

Forgetfulness can be a problem with diaphragms, too,
since they must be inserted prior to intercourse and used in
conjunction with spermicidal jelly or cream. If the dia-

phragm does not fit properly, it is of no use whatsoever. Even properly fitted diaphragms move around during moments of sexual excitation; and the diaphragm must be worn for at least six hours after intercourse, because sperm can remain alive inside the vagina for at least that long.

The very existence of these tough, tiny cells was completely unknown prior to 1677, when Antony van Leeuwenhoek, a Dutch lens grinder, invented the microscope. For reasons best known to him, he examined dog semen under his crude instrument and observed what he called *animalcula*. (Leeuwenhoek was, of course, the first man to see microbes and bacteria, and he shook the scientific community by proving that a drop of ordinary water was teeming with life.) Almost immediately, other scientists began seeking ways to neutralize sperm.

To trace the history of spermicides is to engage in a lengthy and not very interesting history of biochemistry. It is enough for our purposes to recognize that there exist today several spermicides, almost all of which are in the form of creams, jellies, or foams. Some are advertised as sufficiently effective not to require any other contraceptive aid; others are meant to be used in conjunction with diaphragms or cervical caps. All spermicides are applied to the vagina and involve the same risk as any other contraceptive device discussed so far: a spermicide has to be in the right place at the right time. "Accidents," carelessness, or absentmindedness all affect the usefulness of spermicides which, even under ideal conditions, are not 100 percent perfect.

But neutralizing sperm is by no means the only goal to which biochemists dedicated themselves. After long years of testing, experimentation, trial and error, and frustration, science has at last produced an effective oral contraceptive: the Pill.

In the 1880s, medical researchers were beginning to suspect that there is a substance produced in the ovaries that inhibits ovulation, that is, the "positioning" of eggs in the female for fertilization. But it was not until 1934 that the hormone *progesterone* was isolated and recognized as having an effect on ovulation. Not long after, it was discovered that *estrogen* and *testosterone,* also hormones, had similar properties. However, some twenty years elapsed before this information was used to develop an oral contraceptive. Much of the work was done by Dr. Gregory Pincus (who was seeking a contraceptive technique) and by Dr. John Rock (who, ironically, was trying to find a way of increasing fertility). It was not long before the two researchers pooled their resources and information and made some valuable and interesting discoveries.

Basically, it was shown that regular doses of progesterone, estrogen, and testosterone, either singly or in combination, could prevent ovulation. However, the hormones had to be given by extremely painful injections and were very expensive, well beyond the financial reach of the very women who wanted and needed them most. Pincus and Rock worked closely with pharmaceutical laboratories to develop synthetic hormones. Finally, in 1956, a product called Enovid was tested on a large number of women in Puerto Rico.

Although there have been many changes in it since then, the Pill was a reality. It remains for history to show the final effect of this staggering scientific development on Western civilization, but the authors of this book believe that the Pill has already had a tremendous impact on our society and culture. The very foundations of the Judaeo-Christian morality, which has been part of life in America since the landing of the Pilgrims, are being severely shaken. That, however, is a subject for another book (several of which, indeed, have already been written).

To be sure, there are problems with the Pill. Because it is chemical, some women's metabolisms simply cannot tolerate it. Almost all women experience some side effects: a swelling and tenderness of the breasts, slight weight gain, breakthrough bleeding, diminished menstrual flow, and mild nausea in the morning are the most common. Because some of these are the very same symptoms that accompany pregnancy, Pill-takers not alerted to the side effects are confused, to say the least. Diligence is required; one missed day is enough to negate the Pill's effectiveness.

A number of commentators have attempted, without much success, to make a case against the Pill because some women have developed *embolisms*—blood clots—which have proven fatal. But the number is small, and far below the number of women who die in childbirth. Other side effects, while far from dangerous, are nevertheless somewhat disturbing. Some Pill-takers report changes in hair growth, skin condition, urinary regularity, sexual drive, and general mood. It should be remembered that the Pill does consist chiefly of hormones and that upsetting the hormonal balance can, in some women, affect the total organism. Still, as Dr. Selig Neubardt says, "the Pill comes closest to being the ideal contraceptive. Ninety-five out of a hundred women who will give the Pill a try will be completely pleased." [8]

Researchers are still working on an oral contraceptive for men, and according to the rumors and hints that abound, a breakthrough can be expected eventually. One report, unconfirmed, has it that a male pill has actually been developed, but makes the user unable to tolerate alcohol. Another rather disconcerting side effect is that it turns the whites of the eyes purple.

Also in the works, and reputedly very near perfection, is the so-called "morning-after" pill for women. The production of such a pill would make a daily regimen of pill-taking unnecessary. To avoid becoming pregnant, a woman would have to take a pill only on those mornings immediately following intercourse. Technically, she could already be pregnant, assuming that the preceding night's sexual activity caused a sperm cell to fertilize an egg. The morning-after pill, then, is not so much a contraceptive as an *abortifacient* —something that induces an abortion. So is the IUD—the intrauterine device.

For untold centuries, camel drivers have been inserting stones well up inside the vaginas of their female camels to prevent them from becoming pregnant on long journeys (just one more reason why many consider the keeping of camels so unrewarding a way of life). The ignorant, illiterate wanderers of the desert have no idea why this works, but neither do the highly educated, expensively trained scientists who have been studying the same phenomenon in humans.

Apparently, the introduction of a foreign body into the uterus is enough to upset the mechanism that permits a fertilized egg to develop. The egg is dislodged and expelled along with the menstrual fluid. Sometimes, unfortunately, so is the IUD. Dr. Neubardt: "I always recommend the Pill first because it is the most effective and also tends to promote light, regular periods. The coil [IUD] is slightly less effective, may produce heavier than normal periods, and does nothing to correct menstrual irregularity." [9]

Another after-the-fact technique popular through the ages is the douche. But it is almost totally useless. The best that can be hoped for is that no sperm have traveled far or fast enough to cause fertilization before the woman has a chance to douche, and that the douche will reach into all the folds and crevices of the vagina to flush out all the sperm. It helps a little if one of the ingredients of the douche is a spermicide, but some rather exotic fluids have been used from time to time. A home economics teacher in a New York high school told the authors that one of her students confided that the most popular douche among her classmates was warm Coca-Cola. The girl holds her thumb over the open bottle, shakes the contents vigorously, inserts the neck of the bottle in the vagina, removes her finger, and allows the gaseous contents to erupt inside the body. The high rate of pregnancy at the school has done nothing to dispel the popularity of this bit of modern folklore.

It has perhaps not escaped the reader's attention that two important methods—in terms of historical and sociological significance—have so far not been mentioned. They have been saved for last, because they represent the two extremes of contraception: the rhythm method, which is the least effective, and surgical sterilization, which is the most effective.

In 1845, the French Academy of Science awarded its prize for experimental physiology to one Felix Archimedes Pouchet for a report in which he stated that conception in mammals takes place only during menstruation and from one to twelve days following menstruation. The fact that this is completely erroneous and that present-day knowledge is a complete 180-degree turn from Pouchet's more or less summarizes the entire history of the so-called "safe period."

For all practical purposes, a safe period simply does not exist. *Ovulation,* the time when the ovaries place the egg in the most ideal position for fertilization, occurs about two weeks prior to the onset of menstruation, *in general.* So, *if* a couple avoids intercourse for four or five days around that time, and *if* the woman menstruates with clocklike regularity, and *if* nothing happens to upset that regularity —anxiety, a dose of medication, a cold—then perhaps pregnancy can be avoided.

The rhythm method can best be summed up by an old joke:

Question: What do you call people who practice the rhythm method?

Answer: Parents.

What it boils down to is abstinence. If you do not have intercourse—which is what many couples resort to as they expand the "safe period" more and more after the birth of each child—you will avoid pregnancy. Many, including the authors, consider this to be an undue hardship in light of the many contraceptive methods available. If our denunciation of the rhythm method violates certain religious precepts, so be it. We are prepared to accept that responsibility.

Surgical sterilization is unquestionably the most effective method of contraception. It is also probably the least understood. (Some critics also believe it is the most abused, claiming that many hysterectomies—the partial or total removal of the reproductive apparatus of a woman usually because of a tumor—are unnecessary, causing sterility when it is unwanted.) Because of the subject matter of this book, we will touch only lightly on female sterilization.

Two slender tubes—the Fallopian tubes—connect the ovaries with the uterus. These tubes, about the thickness of a toothpick, conduct the egg at ovulation time to a position where it can best be fertilized. Sterilization involves cutting away a small section of each tube and tying off the cut ends. The eggs continue to travel down the Fallopian tubes toward the uterus, but they reach a dead end, where they remain until they are absorbed by the body—a technique the body is quite accustomed to for it continually absorbs used cells that have been replaced by fresh ones. (Keep that in mind; we shall have more to say about it later.)

The operation requires several days' preparation, a general anesthesia, and a small abdominal incision. Because there is some postoperative pain, and because the patient must remain in the hospital for several days, the operation is often performed after the birth of a baby, when the woman must remain in the hospital anyway. After such an operation there is no way in the world she can become pregnant. (Note: See Chapter 1, Question 23.)

Male sterilization is, surgically, a much simpler affair, involving about twenty minutes in the doctor's office, a local anesthetic (such as a shot of Novocaine), and a day or two of relaxing at home. Chances of fathering a child are then absolutely nil. (But not immediately, as shall be explained later.) The entire procedure, step by step, is described in detail in Chapter 4.

Despite the physiological ease with which male sterilization can be accomplished, only a very small percentage of men undergo *vasectomy* (*vas* = duct; *-ectomy* = to cut out). Their reluctance is easy to understand. Sterilization is often equated with loss of manhood, a serious psychological problem that will be fully discussed later on in this book. Much of this feeling stems from the cruel, inhuman, and often dangerous reasons for which knives have been applied to genitalia over the ages. Even at ritual circumcision ceremonies, strong men can be seen to wince when the infant's foreskin is cleanly and surgically removed. (At that, the infant is lucky. Some primitive tribes today do not perform circumcision until the boy has reached puberty.)

Castration, the actual removal of the testicles, does in fact deprive a man of his masculinity—to what extent depends largely upon his age.

Only once in history was castration seen to be a decided advantage. Beginning in the late sixteenth century in Italy (but especially during the seventeenth and eighteenth centuries), if a boy singer had a particularly beautiful voice and if his parents were poor and desperately in need of money, that boy was a likely candidate for becoming a *castrato*. Before his voice changed, the boy was castrated so that he would eventually have the range and tone of a boy soprano or contralto, backed up by the strength and power of a man.

The *castrati* were the darlings of the musical world and, therefore, of the upper classes. Virtually every one of them was extremely wealthy and sought after by women. It became fashionable to have an affair with a *castrato,* presumably because they were so popular (the psychology was no doubt similar to that of the modern rock singer and his "groupies") and because they were "safe."

The last *castrato* died in the early 1900s, but not before recording his voice for posterity. One of the authors has heard that record. Even with the inadequate recording equipment used, it was possible to perceive that his voice was in fact incredibly beautiful. But the price for such beauty was, it seems to us, too high.

Still, there is no connection between vasectomy and castration. Vasectomy causes no loss of manhood, it causes no hormonal changes, it has no effect on one's physical appearance or on one's sex drive. To understand exactly what vasectomy does and does not accomplish, it is necessary to have a fairly good working knowledge of the male sexual apparatus. The next chapter will provide that knowledge.

NOTES

1. Havemann, Ernest: *Birth Control.* New York: Time, Inc., 1967.
2. Suitters, Beryl: *The History of Contraceptives.* London: International Planned Parenthood Federation, 1967.
3. *Webster's Seventh New Collegiate Dictionary.* Springfield, Mass.: G. & C. Merriam Co., 1965.
4. Suitters, Beryl: *op. cit.*
5. Debrovner, Charles H., M.D.: "Sexual and Medical Considerations of Contraception," *Medical Aspects of Human Sexuality,* October 1971.
6. Suitters, Beryl: *op. cit.*
7. *1811 Dictionary of the Vulgar Tongue.* Chicago: Follett Publishing Co., 1971. (Republication of facsimile edition.)
8. Neubardt, Selig, M.D.: *A Concept of Contraception.* New York: Trident Press, 1967.
9. *Ibid.*

3

THE MALE REPRODUCTIVE
SYSTEM

The average layman has only a vague idea of how most of his organs function, both independently and as components in that vast and complex machine which is the human body. It is not surprising; many of the processes and procedures that our organs go through seem nothing short of miraculous and border on the incredible.

The professional anatomists, physiologists, and physicians have not helped by assigning jaw-breaking names to the various parts of the body. There is nothing we can do to simplify the vocabulary, but perhaps we can increase your understanding of what goes on in that relatively small quantity of interestingly arranged flesh, muscle, and tissue which is called the male genitourinary system.

This diagram is a greatly simplified drawing, but it will do nicely. Please refer to it frequently during the rest of this chapter.

First, let us take a quick reconnaissance of the terrain: every high school boy (and most girls, no doubt) knows that sperm, the cells which fertilize the egg in the female after intercourse, are manufactured in the testicles. Through a

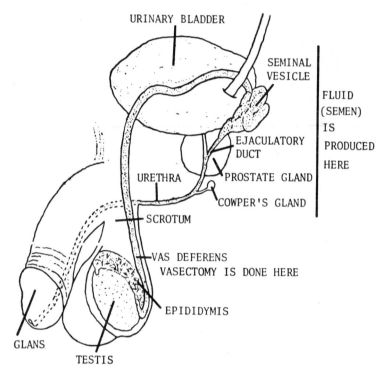

URINARY BLADDER

SEMINAL VESICLE

FLUID (SEMEN) IS PRODUCED HERE

EJACULATORY DUCT

URETHRA

PROSTATE GLAND

COWPER'S GLAND

SCROTUM

VAS DEFERENS
VASECTOMY IS DONE HERE

EPIDIDYMIS

GLANS

TESTIS

SPERM IS PRODUCED HERE

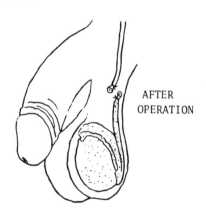

AFTER OPERATION

series of muscular contractions, those sperm are expelled through the erect penis. Stimulus of some kind is required for this to happen. Usually, the stimulant is in the form of friction on the sensitive skin of the penis, but every adult and adolescent male knows that anything from an exciting picture to a half-remembered dream can cause the same result.

Most people know a couple of other things: one is that although liquid body waste (urine) comes out the same place, there is no connection between elimination and the sexual function of the penis. Somehow, the body knows when to urinate and when to ejaculate, and like a railroad switchman, shuts off one to allow the other to pass through. Here is where one of the minor miracles takes place. The bodily functions, essentially mechanical, are triggered by what is happening in and to the psyche. That is why masturbation, for example, is possible. A man can "psych" himself into performing the sex act even when he is not, and his body will respond accordingly. His urinary tract will be shut off and his semen will flow as though he were having sexual intercourse.

Another example of the mind's effect on the body is what happens to you when you see a pretty girl. If she pleases you, the corners of your mouth will go up, without your even being aware of it, and you will be smiling. If she excites you a little, your heart will beat a bit faster, which is not surprising—your penis, about to become erect, is demanding more blood.

Most people also know that the male sex organs are the source of maleness. (The female sex organs, of course, are the source of femaleness.) If for some reason those organs develop abnormally, or if someone "fools around" with them, then their owner will be something less than a man. It is here where most of the psychological problems regarding genital surgery, including vasectomies, arise. And that is why it is important to understand exactly how every component of the male reproductive system works.

Take another look at the diagram. We will start at the very bottom, with the *scrotum.* This is nothing more complicated than a pouch of skin whose sole function is to contain the testicles. But now we begin to get very complicated indeed. Each testicle (or *testis,* as it is often called; plural, *testes*) is a complex little factory. Within that ovate shape, which weighs about half an ounce and measures about three-quarters of an inch thick and an inch-and-a-half long, are packed a thousand threadlike tubes. This is the minuscule chemical factory that produces millions of sperm cells a day. *Testosterone*—the hormone responsible for the depth and timbre of your voice, the hair on your face and chest, the overall shape and musculature of your body; in short, all the obvious and subtle physical characteristics that make you a male—is produced by the so-called Leydig cells in the testes and is passed directly into the bloodstream. *Note: into the bloodstream, and not through any of the other tubes leading from the testes.* Therefore, there are only two ways in which the male chemical testosterone can be prevented from doing its work:

(1) some disease or illness that affects the efficiency of the Leydig cells

(2) the actual removal of the Leydig cells—in other words, the removal of the testes.

Neither of these possibilities is rare or unusual. Cancer, among other diseases, can seriously affect the testes so that they not only cease to function but must be removed. Castration is a frequent result of war. Hazardous occupations, accidents at play—all of these can cause a malfunction of the testes. None of them means the end of masculinity, or even of sexual activity. For one thing, testosterone can be synthesized and taken in sufficient quantities to restore the proper balance. For another, the age of the victim is an important factor. If he is a young boy, the results would be disastrous, because the pubertal changes that depend on testosterone have not yet taken place. But if he is fortyish, there would be very little physical change. Nor would it necessarily interfere with his sexual enjoyment. Many a eunuch, confronted with the tempting ministrations of a neglected denizen of the harem, has been known to rise to the occasion. However, the important thing for a man contemplating vasectomy to remember is that *the vasectomy in no way interferes with the manufacture and distribution of hormones.*

The other important function of the testes is the manufacture of sperm. This too is a highly complicated process. It has no doubt occurred to many a thinking man that if the human body is such a perfect machine, why is it designed so that the testes are *outside,* subject literally to the slings and arrows of fortune, instead of *inside,* where they would be safe and warm? "Warm" is the key word. A temperature three degrees lower than the normal body temperature of 98.6° is required for the manufacture of sperm. (Why this is so is yet another mystery still baffling medical researchers.) So, about two months before birth, the testes drop down through an opening called the inguinal canal, whose only purpose is to allow the passage of the little egg-shapes. Its job done, the inguinal canal closes off. (If it doesn't, the danger of a hernia exists.) But that prenatal descent is by no means the end of the testes' vertical travels, as any man has no doubt observed. When he steps out of a hot shower into a steaming bathroom, the testes hang considerably lower than usual, in an effort to gain greater exposure to the cooling air. If someone suddenly opens the bathroom door and lets a gush of cold air rush in, the scrotum seems to tighten; the testes huddle closer to the body to obtain the warmth needed to maintain constant temperature. The scrotum itself helps out. Its skin is generously packed with sweat glands, providing moisture which hastens cooling when the need to do so arises.

Neither of these manufacturing processes—the making of testosterone or the production of sperm—begins until a boy reaches the age of fourteen or fifteen. Somehow, the pituitary gland, located just under the brain, receives a signal that the teenager is ready, and it triggers the hormonal processes that begin manufacturing sperm and sending testosterone through the bloodstream. The boy's voice changes, he becomes enthralled—and then appalled—with the prospect of having to shave, and those annoying, meddlesome girls suddenly become extremely interesting. How the pituitary knows that the time is right is a secret the gland has yet to reveal. (Pituitary glands are apparently not impressed with changes in culture and the march of progress. When, a scant century or two ago, the average life-span was only forty years, a boy was ready to become a father at the age of fifteen or sixteen, and many of them did just that, with the sanctions and blessings of the society in which they lived.)

The only word for sperm cells is . . . amazing. These tiny tadpolelike structures are similar to no other cell produced in the human body. They contain, among other things, the chromosomes, sticklike chains that help determine the sex and other characteristics (such as the color of eyes and hair) of a man's offspring. All cells contain forty-eight chromosomes, but a sperm holds only twenty-four. The missing half is supplied by the mother's *ovum,* or egg cell. But the tiny sperm, the smallest cell in the entire body, has a long, arduous journey before it can match up its chromosomes with those of a waiting ovum. Let us go back to the diagram and follow it along that journey.

There are two service roads, one emanating from each testis. The road is a long one, and different sections of it have different names. Coming from the starting point, just over the testis, is the *epididymis.* The epididymis is a kind of service station, because in its numerous ducts, the sperm cells receive their *motility,* their power to move forward. *Cilia,* little hairlike projections lining the head of the epididymis, move the sperm along, while the epididymis ducts manufacture the secretion necessary to give the sperm moving power. Musclelike bands around the ducts contract, forcing the secretions into the sperm and moving them along to the starting point. The sperm are now, in effect, ready to roll.

The starting gate is at the beginning of the *vas deferens,* which, from the viewpoint of this book, is the most important part of the entire trip. The vas is a thin, tough tube, about three millimeters in diameter. It looks very much like a thin noodle. Sperm travel along the vas until they reach the *seminal vesicle,* where the *semen,* the thick, milky fluid which makes up most of the ejaculate, is manufactured. The semen's main purpose is to protect the sperm with its alkalinity. There is always a supply of semen in the seminal vesicle—or, almost always. The vesicles are empty, of course, immediately after ejaculation. How long it will take to renew the supply varies from one individual to another. Most sex manuals give an average of a half-hour resting period for recharging, despite the myth of rapid-fire repeat ejaculations so popular in pornography. There are exceptions, but they are very few and very far between.

So far, we have been talking about two paths, one leading from each testicle. Just below the seminal vesicle is the *ejaculatory duct,* the entrance to the *urethra,* which will be discussed in a moment. Just under the crossroads of the ejaculatory duct is the *prostate,* a word that conjures up fear in most men. The prostate is a gland that secretes nutrients, antacids, and enzymes for the sperm, but its role is not essential. Most men can function without it. When a man reaches fifty years of age, or thereabout, it is a good idea to have the prostate checked regularly because it can become inflamed, enlarged, infected, or a source of malignancy. When any of those things happen, urination becomes difficult, sometimes painful, and often, in severe cases, impossible, leading to infection. Fortunately a malfunctioning prostate is easily removed by surgery.

The *urethra* is a long tube that originates in the bladder and extends to the end of the penis. It is through this tube that both semen and urine pass. Along the way, the sperm, now carried in the seminal fluid, pick up a little lubrication from the Cowper's gland.

The purpose of the *penis* is to deposit the sperm-laden semen deep inside the vagina. The best way for this to be accomplished is for the penis to be erect, and it is superbly engineered for that purpose.

The penis is comprised primarily of two long columns of muscle tissue called *corpora cavernosa.* These muscles are heavily interlaced with blood vessels, which are empty most of the time. When a man becomes sexually aroused, the brain signals the penis that the sex act is about to occur. (Like the pituitary, the brain and penis are unconcerned with morals and rules; those belong to the province of the mind.) Blood rapidly fills the normally relaxed vessels, causing the penis to become stiff and hard. When that happens, you can easily feel, along the back of the penis, the *corpus spongiosum,* a third, smaller muscular column that contains the urethra.

Now, let us return to the testis and follow the sperm on their journey. The penis has become sexually aroused and the *corpora cavernosa* becomes filled with blood. During intercourse, the penis becomes increasingly stimulated until orgasm. At this point, here is what happens:

Sperm move from the testes into the epididymis where they are infused with their motile power. They then move into the vas deferens, stop at the seminal vesicles just long enough to pick up the seminal fluid, receive a little shot from the prostate, another little shot from the Cowper's gland, and in a series of involuntary muscular spasms, the whole rich mixture spurts through the urethra and out of the penis—all in less time than it takes to read this last sentence!

The journey for the sperm cells is by no means over. There is still a long, hazardous trip to be made inside the female genitalia, but that is another story.

If this was the first ejaculation in a twenty-four-hour period, the semen could contain about a hundred million sperm cells. Yet if those cells were not there, neither partner would be aware of any difference in the quantity of fluid ejaculated. Sperm make up about 5 percent of the total ejaculate. The period at the end of this sentence represents the space occupied by over a thousand sperm cells.

If the testes do not have a chance to manufacture fresh supplies, the sperm count can become rather low after the first few ejaculations. But supposing the penis is not stimulated for a relatively long period of time. What happens to the sperm cells being stored in the body?

They die. Human cells die all the time. When you take a bath, some of the film that forms on top of the bath water is dead skin cells. The body is continually manufacturing fresh, healthy cells to replace the used, worn-out ones. When this happens internally, the dead cells are absorbed into the bloodstream and eventually passed out of the body with waste.

Precisely the same thing happens to sperm cells. If you go for a long period of time without an orgasm, the sperm cells in your body will die. The dead cells will be replaced with new, fresh, live ones. Your bloodstream will convey the dead cells to points where they can be eliminated from the body (through urination, defecation, perspiration). This is more than merely a natural process; it is the essence of staying alive. Death occurs when the body is no longer capable of removing old cells and replacing them with new ones. This is extremely important to remember, because this removal-and-replacement process is what happens to unused sperm cells after a vasectomy.

Now, let's see how a vasectomy is performed.

4

THE VASECTOMY

The best time to have a vasectomy performed is on a Friday afternoon, and in fact the vast majority of these operations takes place at that time. This gives the patient the entire weekend to recuperate, although in most cases he does not need that much time.

We are now going to assume that a fictitious patient, Harry, has decided to have a vasectomy. Let's follow him, step by step, through the procedure.

Harry has made an appointment with his physician, Dr. Fletcher, but prior to that the doctor counseled him on all the pros and cons. Presumably, Harry will have been given at least as much information as you will have by the time you finish this book. In addition, the doctor will have taken into account certain personal aspects of Harry's marriage, family situation, and life-style. (More about this in the next chapter.)

Certain preliminaries will have been gone through in advance of the operation. Harry will have been given a general physical examination to be sure he is in good health. Dr. Fletcher will want to be certain that Harry has no blood

51

disease or uncontrolled blood sugar. His urine will also be analyzed. Most important, Dr. Fletcher will want to take a sperm count before he even seriously considers surgery.

You will recall that sperm are the smallest cells the body produces. Therefore, the microscope provides the only means of determining whether Harry is in fact fertile. (Of course, another way to tell is for Harry to make someone pregnant, but that seems a trifle extreme just to determine the viability of his sperm when a simple laboratory procedure will do the job just as well.) So Harry will provide Dr. Fletcher with a semen specimen. This can be done in two ways: Harry can have regular sexual intercourse with his wife. Just as he is about to reach orgasm, he withdraws and ejaculates into a clean glass bottle. The other method is for Harry to masturbate, either at home or in a private room at the doctor's office, again ejaculating into a clean glass container. Despite the difficulty some men may have reaching orgasm under such clinical conditions, the latter method is preferred. Sperm are very sensitive to changes in temperature, and if Harry "comes" at home, he will not only have to get the specimen to the doctor within an hour or two, but he will also have to keep it warm.

The physician will then examine Harry's sperm under a microscope. He will check for three things: quantity, quality, and motility. If the actual count—the sperm population, as it were—of Harry's semen is extremely low, the physician may well recommend that the vasectomy not be performed, because Harry's chances of impregnating his wife are very slim. If there are no sperm at all, then Harry is already sterile.

A normal, healthy sperm looks like a slightly egg-shaped head, to which is attached a long, thin tail. If the vast majority of sperm cells in Harry's semen fails to conform to this description, then for all practical purposes he is sterile. Sperm with short or missing tails, tails that are all curled or twisted, heads that are misshapen, are all ill-equipped to make that tortuous journey through the vagina and into the uterus to fertilize an egg.

Everything for which a sperm cell is designed and intended depends upon its ability to move. The doctor will check very carefully, therefore, for motility; even if Harry's sperm are as plentiful as grains of sand on the beach, and their form and shape are as gorgeous as one could hope for, they are useless if they are not good swimmers. That is why it is imperative that Harry's semen specimen be brought in quickly and that it be kept warm. Time and temperature can kill motile sperm and give a wrong impression of their original liveliness. As part of his test for motility, Dr. Fletcher will carefully note the direction in which the sperm are moving. If they seem to be swimming about willy-nilly with no particular destination in mind, then for all practical purposes the sperm have low or no motility. If they are all heading more or less in one direction, then they have viable motility.

If Harry's sperm failed to pass any one of these tests— quantity, quality, motility—then a vasectomy is not indicated. Should Harry protest that he already has children, then there are three possibilities to consider: (1) Harry is a very lucky man whose sperm cells have managed, against all odds, to reach their destination; (2) some ailment or drastic change in Harry's life has brought about a change in his sperm and this change occurred after his children were born; (3) Harry's wife is a very sociable woman.

As it happens, Dr. Fletcher has informed Harry that all systems are go and the appointment has been made for the operation to be performed in the doctor's office. The great majority of vasectomies are done this way. A relatively few physicians still feel more comfortable performing surgery of any kind in a hospital, and among them there are some who prefer a general anesthetic (i.e., one that puts the patient to sleep for a period of time) to a local anesthetic (one that deadens all sensation in a given area). If Harry were a particularly squeamish type, Dr. Fletcher would have recommended a general anesthetic, and this would automatically mean that Harry would have to be hospitalized. But as it turns out, the only thing Harry is squeamish about is shaving.

Dr. Fletcher advised Harry that he would have to shave his pubic hair, and most particularly, the hair on his scrotum. Already a little nervous about having the skilled hands of the surgeon using a blade on his genitals, Harry is absolutely petrified over the prospect of shaving between his legs. Fletcher told Harry not to worry; he would take care of it. To Harry's dismay, he learns too late that Fletcher was only partly telling the truth. Stretched out on the table, his feet up in stirrups, Harry discovers that Dr. Fletcher's idea of taking care of something like this is to have his nurse do it! Blushing the full length of his body, Harry closes his eyes and grits his teeth, while his good sense tries to break through his embarrassment to inform him that the nurse has seen and handled more male genitalia in a week than the average woman does in an entire lifetime. Anyway, by the time Harry has reconciled himself to the situation and is in fact beginning to enjoy it a little, the job is done. The next step is a thorough washing with a medically approved detergent. Then an antiseptic, usually aqueous Zephiran or a similar product, is painted over the scrotum. The entire area, except for the scrotum, is covered with sterile drapes.

Carefully and gently, Dr. Fletcher feels for the vas through the skin of the scrotum and holds it between his thumb and index finger. Actually, what he is holding is the *spermatic cord*. In our last chapter, for purposes of simplification, we treated the vas as though it were completely independent and separate. In fact, however, the vas is encased in the spermatic cord, a kind of coaxial cable that also contains blood vessels, muscle layers, and mucous membrane.

Now, with his other hand, Dr. Fletcher injects a small quantity of local anesthetic, usually some form of Novocaine. This will eliminate all feeling in the scrotal area long enough for Dr. Fletcher to perform the surgery. When he has determined that Harry will feel no pain, the doctor makes a tiny incision—about one-half to three-quarters of an inch in length—in the scrotum. The spermatic cord is now grasped with forceps and lifted out through the incision. Another pair of forceps is placed under it to hold it in place.

A little more Novocaine is injected, this time into the spermatic cord itself. A small incision is made in the cord, and the vas deferens is pulled out. Two clamps are placed an inch apart on the vas. A one-inch segment of the vas is removed, and the cut ends are securely tied with catgut sutures.

Dr. Fletcher—and the medical coauthor of this book—perform the actual vasectomy as has just been described. (For the purists, we should point out that the "vasectomy," as has been clearly shown by the preceding paragraph, is a misnomer. Technically speaking, "partial vasectomy" is more accurate because only a part of the vas is removed.) Many physicians, however, use other techniques. Some do not remove a section of the vas. Instead, they make a single cut and then fold the ends back on themselves. The theory behind this is that should the patient later decide to have the operation reversed, it is easier to do so—although it may also be pointless to do so, as we shall discuss in Chapter 9. Another method is to *cauterize* the cut ends, that is, seal them up with scar tissue by burning them slightly. Each method is equally effective and is largely a matter of personal preference on the part of the surgeon.

Harry's vas has just been cut and tied. It is now allowed to slip back into the spermatic cord, and the cord slides back into the scrotum. A single stitch, sometimes two, closes the incision in the scrotum. Dr. Fletcher sprinkles the wound with an antibiotic powder and then he goes to the other side of the table and does the same thing all over again to the other vas.

Twenty minutes after the first incision was made, Harry is ready to sit up and, after putting on a scrotal support—a kind of light jockstrap—he can go home.

Admittedly, not every case is as easy as Harry's. Sometimes a vas is difficult to locate. On occasion, a patient has a tendency to bleed a little heavily. Every now and then, the doctor can find only one vas because the patient *has* only one vas. All of these occurrences can extend the operating time to as long as forty-five minutes. But the average vasectomy takes from twenty to thirty minutes.

Harry may be out of the operating room, but he is not out of the woods. For one thing, he is not yet sterile (more about that shortly). For another, the Novocaine has not worn off yet. When it does, he can expect to feel some aftereffects.

There will no doubt be a little pain when the anesthetic wears off. A couple of aspirins should take care of it, but if it gets to be really bad, Harry should call Dr. Fletcher and let him know. There may also be a little bleeding, especially if one of the stitches comes loose, but this too will subside in most cases. If it persists, again Dr. Fletcher should be notified.

About the best thing for Harry to do is to go home and

watch TV or read for the rest of the day. By the following morning he can resume virtually all his normal activities, including work, as long as he does not engage in anything strenuous. It might be a good idea, for example, to forego his usual Sunday morning golf game for just this once. Horseback riding and bicycling are also ill-advised, as are crowds, where he might be jostled. By the following weekend, however, Harry can do pretty much as he chooses.

He can begin bathing or showering the day after the operation, as long as he washes the genital area gently and blots it dry instead of rubbing it. The stitches will dissolve by themselves, and Harry should wear the supporter until the incision heals and the stitches have disappeared.

A few men—very few—do suffer from other side effects. One of the more common is a mild state of depression, but it is not a genuine cause for concern. Almost any kind of *trauma* (i.e., unusual occurrence) to the body, even the common cold, can cause depression. Some dentists, for example, have learned to their dismay that a dose of Novocaine can cause a patient to have a crying jag.

Other unusual side effects of vasectomy can be more serious. In 1969 the Simon Population Trust, which operates a vasectomy clinic in Cambridge, England, conducted one of the most extensive surveys ever made among vasectomized men. They interviewed 1012 men and learned, among other things, that "of 326 men who reported disagreeable aftereffects, thirty-three merited serious attention." These included postoperative infection and *hematomata,* the formation of blood clots. One man had scrotal swelling, another a testicular swelling. Four experienced *epididymitis,* inflammation of the epididymis. "These thirty-three men who mentioned aftereffects which called for attention constitute a small minority of 3.1 percent which should be compared with the majority of over two-thirds (67 percent) who suffered no aftereffects." The remaining 293 reports of aftereffects were "mostly, medically speaking, trivial [and called] for little or no time off [from work]." [1] Even distress of the very few who could be considered moderately serious does not compare with the seriousness of an unwanted pregnancy.

But the big question in Harry's mind (and in yours, too, no doubt) is sex. Has the operation changed Harry? Is he less of a man now? Is he sterile? The answers are no, no, and no. Harry is not changed in any way. Once his pubic hair has grown out, he looks, acts, and feels exactly as he did before the vasectomy. Harry feels confident, self-assured, and pleased with himself because he knows that soon an unwanted pregnancy will never again be a problem for him and his wife. He knows that his manhood has not been affected in any way because the surgery did not have anything to do with his testicles. They will continue to manufacture the male hormones which give Harry his masculinity, and those hormones are passing into his bloodstream in exactly the same way they have been doing ever since he was fourteen. In fact, immediately after the operation, even Harry's fertility is exactly the same! If Harry thinks he is sterile, he is making a very serious error.

Harry can resume normal intercourse with his wife within four or five days after the vasectomy, but he must use the same contraceptive techniques he has been relying on all along. Before he can forget about contraception, it will take Harry several ejaculations to remove all the remaining sperm from his genital plumbing, from the point the vas is cut to the opening of his urethra. Just how long it will take varies from man to man. It may be as few as two or three ejaculations; there have been reports of viable sperm remaining after twenty-five ejaculations. Dr. Fletcher has told Harry to return with a semen specimen after four ejaculations. If he finds live sperm, he will advise Harry to continue using contraceptives and to return with a semen specimen after three more ejaculations. Harry will have to keep coming back until Dr. Fletcher finds that the semen is completely clear of sperm. And on that happy day, Harry can throw away his condoms, his wife can throw out her diaphragm and get rid of her Pills. Harry is now sterile, and unwanted babies are no longer a factor in his life.

Under normal circumstances, most vasectomy patients require no more than two semen examinations after the operation. But on rare occasions the doctor continues to find viable sperm in the semen. Clearly, something has gone wrong. The vasectomy has failed.

In ninety-nine out of a hundred cases, vasectomy "failure" is the fault of the patient, who quickly becomes impatient. He cannot be bothered with return trips to the physician for sperm counts and yet he is surprised when, shortly after the operation, his wife becomes pregnant again. This cannot be regarded as a surgical failure because the father-to-be will eventually become sterile when his genital tubes and ducts become free of sperm. It may be a medical failure if his physician has neglected to impress upon him the necessity of subsequent semen examinations.

On rare occasions a vasectomized man may experience *spontaneous reanastomosis*—the tendency the body has to make itself whole again. There is a kind of built-in biological urge for the separated ends of the vas to get together and bridge the gap. When vasectomy is performed by actually removing a portion of the vas, reanastomosis will almost never occur. Despite the extreme rarity of reanastomosis, some authorities recommend that vasectomized men return for a sperm count as much as a year after the operation. In

England, according to a recent *New York Times* article, it is possible to take out an insurance policy against pregnancy after vasectomy. The article states that "according to an insurance reference work, 'Excess and Surplus Lines Manual,' in order to collect, 'there must be evidence that the husband had a positive sperm count after the pregnancy.' " [2] (The policy evidently insures against impatience, surgical failure, and spontaneous reanastomosis, but not against hanky-panky.)

Surgically, there is only one reason for vasectomy failure: failure to interrupt the continuity of the vas. Obviously, if the surgeon cuts the wrong tube, the operation has been worse than useless.

But useless is not hopeless. As a matter of course, the surgeon will send the excised portion of the vas to a pathologist for confirmed identification of the structure and for what doctors refer to as any "subtle pathology" of the vas. In other words, the pathology laboratory's report will confirm that the proper plumbing has been attended to and will also reveal any problems of a medical nature that may have existed unknown to the patient or the doctor.

Finding a competent physician who will perform a vasectomy is not easy. But it is not impossible, either, once you know how, as we shall discuss in the next chapter.

NOTES

1. "Vasectomy: Follow-up of a Thousand Cases," report by The Simon Population Trust, Cambridge, England, December 1969.
2. Cole, Robert J.: " 'Kooky' Insurance," *The New York Times,* April 2, 1972.

5

YOU AND YOUR DOCTOR

Sometimes in the mass media, but more often in private conversations, doctors are accused of harboring self-images bordering on godliness. Like most extreme statements, these accusations contain a kernel of truth. But it is this very truth that gives evidence that far from being above reproach, doctors are very human indeed—because those who feel that they are something special are usually made to feel so by their patients. What can be a more human failing than responding to the idolization and admiration of our fellow man?

Still, one should remember that no matter how skilled, competent, and successful a physician may be in his profession, he is only a human being. It is as important for the patient to remember this as it is for the doctor. A doctor has a personality; he is subject to moods, tempers, tantrums, and spells; he has a religion (which may be atheism); he has a moral code that has absolutely nothing to do with his professional skill but which nevertheless affects his professional practice; he has prejudices and weaknesses; he has impartialities and strengths. In short, he has all the components that make up the whole man—just as you do. In an era when skilled medical practitioners are scarce, it can be extremely difficult for a patient to find a physician whose view of the world is the same as his own. And indeed, in most instances, particularly where a specialist is concerned, there is no real need to do so. After all, if you suffer a broken leg, it makes no real difference whether the orthopedist who sets it is a Republican or a Democrat, or whether he believes marijuana should be legalized.

But we are not talking about broken bones. We are talking about voluntary sterilization, the deliberate alteration of one of the human body's most basic functions. It is frequently forgotten that voluntary sterilization involves a voluntary act not only on the patient's part, but on the surgeon's as well. How the surgeon reacts to his role in the matter varies widely from individual to individual. There are many physicians who feel that any "tampering" with the body is unethical or immoral if it is not required for pathological reasons. There are, however, just as many who believe they are morally and professionally bound to "improve" the body whenever possible. (If this were not so, cosmetic "plastic" surgery would not enjoy its current popularity.) Yet, one would be hard pressed to locate, for example, a surgeon who would perform an appendectomy as a deterrent against possible future appendicitis (except, perhaps, in the course of other abdominal surgery).

To the differences that exist between the "antitampering" school and the "improvement" school must be added those that arise from philosophical considerations. Some say every man has the right to determine what to do with his own body, up to and including suicide. Their opposite numbers claim that only God or Nature has the right to pass such judgment, and that while it is the doctor's duty to preserve health and life, no man has the right to defy a set pattern of morals and ethics, even though such defiance involves only his own body and seemingly has no effect on anyone else.

These arguments get really complex as soon as sex enters the picture. So much has been said and written about the morality of sex that it becomes an integral part of everyone's view of life. Doctors are no exception. Many physicians are as confused, pleased, angered, envious, applauding, and condemning of the so-called new morality as are most laymen. It is impossible for any physician—unless he is that rare individual who does indeed approach godliness—to divorce his personal feelings, many of which may be unconscious, from his professional practice, especially when it comes to something like vasectomies.

There is general agreement that any physician who is asked to perform a vasectomy has a moral and ethical obligation to counsel his patient about the operation. It is in that counseling that the doctor's own personality and his outlook on life become critical.

Dr. Robert B. Benjamin, a prominent surgeon, writes: "In counseling couples who are considering vasectomy as a means of contraception, I have tried to play the role of resource person rather than judge. I believe the surgeon should refrain from making value judgments or decisions such as 'you are *too young* to have a vasectomy' or 'you *do not have enough children.*' "[1]

Is Dr. Benjamin's attitude right? It all depends on which doctor you talk to. The value judgments he eschews are among the very ones that many doctors take into consideration. Let's examine some of them.

Age of patient. Many surgeons will simply refuse to perform a vasectomy on any man under the age of twenty-five, regardless of any other considerations. Most who hold to this restriction will make exceptions in cases where the patient is a low-income father of four or five children. As a matter of fact, Dr. Helen Edey, a psychiatrist whom we shall get to know better later on in this book, offers some good reasons for not performing vasectomies on younger men, but they are psychological reasons having to do with the patient rather than with the physician. (We'll go into those reasons in the next chapter.)

Marital status. A great many doctors will not perform vasectomies on unmarried men, regardless of how much the would-be patient pleads for it or is willing to pay. They feel that a single man who wants to become sterile is probably a "swinger" or has ambitions of becoming one, and they will not contribute to such behavior, which they consider immoral.

This is a perfect example of a physician's personal morals influencing his professional practice. Should a man, single or married, have the right to do as he chooses with his own body? Does the physician have the right to pass moral judgment? Does not the physician have the obligation and the responsibility of preserving a high moral level in our society? The answers to these questions vary, depending on the particular doctor you happen to be talking to.

Marital stability. How involved should the doctor become in the personal lives of his patients? His obvious obligation is to inform the patient of all physiological consequences of the surgery, but should he ask questions or seek insights into the marital stability of the patient? After all, how much can a surgeon be held responsible for?

Dr. Edey lays the responsibility squarely on the shoulders of the physician. "It is perfectly true," she says, "that the fear of pregnancy may inhibit sexual enjoyment and reduce its frequency. But any hope in either spouse for a magic cure of sexual problems must be extinguished by the doctor before surgery." [2] All well and good. But such false hopes cannot be "extinguished" unless they are discovered, and they can only be discovered by digging for them. Again, a two-sided argument arises. On the one hand, the doctor may be seen to have an obligation to dispel false hopes. On the other, a surgeon can no more be expected to perform "quickie" psychoanalysis than a psychiatrist can be expected to perform "quickie" surgery.

Perhaps between these two extremes is the experienced, mature practitioner who has been around people long enough to recognize an up-tight psyche when he meets one. More than one surgeon has recommended psychiatry before vasectomy.

Law. Vasectomies are now legal in all fifty states. Furthermore, no physician will perform the operation without a written consent signed by both the husband and wife. (A typical release form will be found in Appendix A.) If the wife shows any reluctance at all, most doctors will not operate.

There is a good psychological reason, from the couples' point of view, for not operating in such instances, but in many cases—and quite justifiably—the doctor is thinking of himself first. If the wife is not thoroughly convinced that a vasectomy for her husband is a good thing, she can very quickly transform herself into a big problem that goes by the name of Malpractice Suit. Despite the reassurances from medical journals that such suits have almost no chance of succeeding, most doctors are cautious. Who can blame them?

Religion. Orthodox Jews and Muslims, and practicing Roman Catholics, are opposed to birth control of any kind. "Obviously," editorializes the American Medical Association in its *Journal,* "the Catholic physician and the Catholic patient must resolve any medico-religious conflicts in accord with their own consciences and beliefs. But the rest of the country must not be deprived of a legitimate method of contraception because of the opposition of any outside group." [3] That is not as easy as it sounds. For one thing, many Catholic surgeons, perfectly capable of performing voluntary vasectomies, may simply refuse to do so, despite the AMA's injunctions against influence by an "outside group." A would-be patient who inadvertently goes to a Catholic physician may get a sermon instead of surgery.

Because of the traditional Jewish attitudes against proselytizing, an Orthodox Jewish doctor may cheerfully vasectomize any non-Jew who asks for it, while considering it his religious obligation to try to convince his Jewish patients against it. Furthermore, if the Catholic, Orthodox Jewish, or Muslim physician has deep religious convictions against sterilization, those beliefs may affect his "counseling" of patients, including those who are not coreligionists.

Even the AMA, in its attempt at objectivity, slips in a value judgment. The same editorial quoted above concludes: ". . . If a man can reconcile the operation with his religion: *if he has several children*; if he lacks observable psychiatric sex-oriented stigmata; and if his wife agrees to the operation—surely, then, he should be able to obtain a vasectomy for reasons of contraception alone." [4] (Italics added.) The need for wifely consent and for the absence of "psychiatric sex-oriented stigmata" are fairly obvious; they represent medical and legal considerations. Does the presence of "several children" represent a moral consideration, a value judgment? The answer to that question is again a value judgment in itself, which each physician must—and does—make for himself.

If patients tend to regard physicians as purely objective,

suprahuman scientists, other physicians do not. Dr. Edey advises that "a doctor should not project onto the patient his own subjective weighing of the various factors, his own feelings about having children, his own sexual anxiety, or his own satisfaction with other contraceptive methods." [5] She recognizes that what doctors *should not* do and what they *do not* do are often two different things. In another paper, she observes: "Men confuse sterilization with castration, and even if reassured, many cannot resolve this anxiety. I believe that male doctors are not immune to this problem." [6] Among the things most patients expect from their doctors is a sizable dose of reassurance. It is hard to come by, however, if the doctor has his own hangups about the treatment he is giving.

We believe that in expecting the medical profession to do more than perform medically, many doctors are asking too much of their colleagues. It is our conviction that reassurance, founded on knowledge, is primarily the patient's responsibility, bolstered and supported by information from the concerned medical practitioner. Anyone considering a vasectomy should regard his physician essentially as an expert who can perform tasks that the patient cannot perform himself. Thus, the patient's first consideration in seeking out a surgeon is to find one whose skills are proven.

Probably any surgeon can perform a vasectomy, but it is generally recommended that the operation be performed by a *urologist,* a doctor whose specialty is the genitourinary system, as he is likely to have extensive experience in vasectomies, including any complications that may arise. At the risk of alienating some interns and residents, we recommend a urologist who has been around for a while, for nothing replaces experience. As one doctor put it, ". . . good surgical technique and repetition with the procedure will prevail to mold the novice into an accomplished office vasectomist with a track time usually depending on the condition of the turf." [7]

If you do not know a urologist, there are several ways to find one. Your family physician, or any specialist you may have dealt with, probably knows one he can recommend to you. Your county or state medical association will also recommend several, usually with some effort to maintain impartiality. The New York County Medical Society, for example, will recommend three physicians in any specialization who are members of the Society, chosen at random. Most other medical associations have similar procedures.

The nearest office of any group concerned with population control will refer you to doctors who perform vasectomies. Perhaps the easiest way to locate a physician for vasectomy is to write or telephone the Association for Voluntary Sterilization, Inc., 14 W. 40th St., New York, N.Y. 10018; telephone (212) 524–2344.

If you prefer a clinic or a hospital to a private doctor, Appendix B lists vasectomy clinics and hospitals where vasectomies are performed as an out-patient procedure.

As a matter of course, many people often check out a new doctor whose name is not accompanied by a high personal recommendation. Most public libraries have directories of local physicians, giving their qualifications: education, specialties, hospital affiliations, societies, honors, etc. A few minutes spent in wading through the tedious technical abbreviations are rewarded by a good deal of added confidence in the doctor.

Confidence in the doctor, engendered by a knowledge of his background and his experience, and an understanding of his potential hangups, is important. But even more important is confidence in yourself and an understanding of *your* potential hangups. Having examined the doctor, let's now have a close look at the patient.

NOTES

1. Benjamin, Robert B., M.D.: "Vasectomy as an Office Procedure," *The Bulletin,* St. Louis Park Medical Center, Vol. XIV, No. 1, winter quarter 1970.
2. Edey, Helen M., M.D.: "Psychological Aspects of Vasectomy," *Vasectomy,* "presented by the Center for the Advancement of Population Studies in Medicine and the Student American Medical Association, Ecology Committee," 1972.
3. American Medical Association: "Voluntary Male Sterilization" (editorial) *Journal,* May 27, 1968.
4. *Ibid.*
5. Edey, Helen M.: *op. cit.*
6. Edey, Helen M., M.D.: "Sterilization," *New York Medicine,* August 1970.
7. Fadil, Richard, M.D., F.A.C.S.: "Vasectomies: Hospital or Office?" *Vasectomy* (see Note 2).

6

THE MACHISMO FACTOR

But then comes the psychological crunch, the most deeply-rooted fear of all. Whisper it: castration. Vasectomy is not castration. But symbolic or actual, virtually all men, whatever their sexual inclinations, carry that piece of emotional baggage around in their psyche. Not everyone can work it out.[1]

The key to that paragraph, which appeared as part of a recent magazine article, is in the phrase "symbolic or actual." Even among men who fully understand that "vasectomy is *not* castration," the fear, or at least the association, still lurks.

In an important study conducted in 1967 among seventy-three vasectomized men and their wives, the researchers felt that "vasectomy does stimulate infantile fears and fantasies of castration, impotence, and concomitant decline in self-esteem." [2] (The full title of this study, and its authors, can be found in the note at the end of the chapter. We will refer to the study as the FTL Study, for authors Ferber, Tietze, and Lewit.) Still, education does seem to be a factor, and while more and more so-called blue-collar workers are undergoing the operation, at least one physician has noted "the strong impression that the highly educated, well-to-do Caucasian is more likely to request vasectomy than the less educated, poor member of a minority racial group. An inordinately high percentage of physicians, ministers, social workers, professors, teachers, and lawyers are found among those who have undergone vasectomy in my practice." [3] This is, of course, one doctor's practice, but indications are not very different among the physicians we have talked to. On the other hand, some of the vasectomy clinics are reporting a slight but growing increase in lower-income and minority-group patients, although none is willing to give statistics yet.

(Part of the problem in studying the whole subject of voluntary sterilization is that studies and surveys seem to be conducted somewhat sporadically. But with 750,000 men having been vasectomized in the United States in 1970 and another 800,000 in 1971—with estimates for a million more in 1972—it appears likely that new studies will soon be forthcoming.)

Part of the reason for associating vasectomy with castration may have to do with simple ignorance, which can be corrected merely by informing the ignorant of the facts. But that would solve only part of the problem, because the fear persists even among the educated. The FTL Study concluded that "vasectomy is perceived by all men, on some level, in some way, as a castration." [4] Different men have different ways of coping with the problem.

Jim Bouton, former baseball star, a best-selling author, and now a sports commentator, related, in a conversation with the authors: "In spite of what I had read about it, I insisted on a local anesthetic. I wanted to keep an eye on the guy with the knife. If it was everything he said it was, fine, but I didn't want to wake up surprised." A completely different attitude was expressed by writer Bailey Alexander: "One of my most persistent images had me strapped to the operating table, the surgeon's knife poised . . . and a playful nurse goosing the doctor at a highly critical point in the proceedings. When that particular fantasy first materialized, I knew I would insist upon total anesthesia during the operation. I wasn't about to be awake in the event my most cherished possession was accidentally snipped off like a wilted geranium." [5]

Neither of these two completely different methods of coping with the same fear resolves the fact that the fear is essentially unfounded. If a doctor were to castrate a man, he would have to do so deliberately. The surgeon uses a small scalpel for vasectomy; he does not use a meat axe or a pair of garden shears. Even if he were to "slip"—a highly unlikely possibility—the damage, if any, would be slight. Certainly castration would not be the result of such a slip. But this argument is founded on logic and reason, neither of which has very much impact on deeply embedded emotions. Dr. Edey described these emotions in a personal interview: "There is the unconscious anxiety about their own true masculinity. . . . They feel they are going to be so anxious after the operation about whether they really are potent that they will indeed get themselves into a condition of having sexual problems.

"A lot of men," she explained, "are unconsciously very insecure about their masculinity. They're not saying to themselves, 'Let's see, I'm insecure about my masculinity so I may work myself into something.' But they are unconsciously very insecure about [it], and anything which reverberates in their minds as a threat, or which at some point in their lives they have felt as a threat, reawakens the insecurity and they just can't accept this hypothetical threat even if their knowledge tells them it isn't there."

In other words, men with sexual hangups should probably not have vasectomies. There is, as a matter of fact, a certain self-selection: the primary reason such a high percentage of vasectomized men are pleased with the results is that they are free of the kinds of problems that a vasectomy would tend to deepen. Men who do have such problems do not as a rule have vasectomies. When they do, almost certain emotional disaster is the result, as we shall soon see.

But even among men who seem to have reconciled these problems and are quite convinced that there is no relationship between vasectomy and loss of manhood, there is a reluctance to discuss the operation with others. "It seemed clear," the FTL Study reported, "that most men assumed a loss of status attendant upon sterilization, and while willing to deal with their own internal self-critique, were reluctant to face the disapproval of others." [6] Jim Bouton, who had his vasectomy in 1969, told us: "Some friends of mine were stunned when they heard I was going to get a vasectomy. People don't know what it is; they think you're being castrated or deformed." The authors found, in an informal survey, that many vasectomized men are particularly reluctant to discuss the operation with their parents and in-laws, claiming, as one patient put it, "They would never understand."

Fortunately, this attitude seems to be undergoing a gradual but noticeable change. In the interview, Dr. Edey related an interesting situation at the Margaret Sanger Bureau, in New York, where she counsels all vasectomy applicants.

"I remember after we had been there about three months, a policeman came in and he said he wasn't going to tell anybody he knew. But strangely enough, two months later we had another policeman from the same precinct, and then another few, and before too long it seemed to me that practically the entire precinct had come in.

"The police department," she added, "has been flooding into Margaret Sanger. Now we're starting on firemen and sanitation workers." Apparently, these public servants, with whose work masculinity is always associated, have no fears about their effectiveness as men. The fact that GHI, a popular health insurance plan among government workers, covers vasectomies (as do most health plans, by the way) may have had some small influence.

Sometimes, "the unconscious anxiety about their own true masculinity" to which Dr. Edey refers manifests itself in a manner which, on the surface, seems to indicate exactly the opposite. Almost everyone knows the "Don Juan" or "lady-killer" type who carves notches on his bedpost the way Wild West gunslingers used to cut them on their pistols. When a man makes a career of bedding down every female who will submit to his enticements, when he keeps score by numbers yet finds difficulty in establishing a deep relationship with any one woman, it is a fairly safe bet that deep in his psyche he harbors some fear either about sex or about his own sexual abilities. He makes love not because he enjoys doing so but because he has to "prove" that his unconscious fears and doubts are unfounded. A vasectomy for such a man could be a boon, providing him with the ability to fill the void in his psyche with greater ease. On the other hand, it could also be calamitous: his lack of sexual self-confidence could be worsened by the knowledge that he is sterile. In any event, such a man is likely to be unmarried, and the general consensus among the experts is that unmarried men should not be vasectomized in the first place.

According to Dr. Edey, "the man should have had sufficient experience to be able to truly imagine the consequences of his act, the possibility of chance in himself or his circumstances, and a certain range of emotions. In this experience, opportunities for a lasting relationship with a woman should be included. To be more blunt, I do not believe that single young men under twenty-four or twenty-five generally have had this range of experience. I find them rather unimaginative. . . ." [7]

Along these same lines, Dr. Edey said during the interview: "In truth, [the single man under twenty-five] simply lacks the imagination to realize how changeable he is, how he'll feel when he's married to a woman he cares about and who wants a baby. When I talk to him he often does seem to have a great lack of imagination. He seems to be fixed on certain life-styles he's convinced will never change, yet he's uncertain as to what he will do with his life."

In Chapter 9, we will discuss why vasectomies should be considered 100 percent irreversible (although this is not exactly so). Because it can be, and often is, a final step with no turning back, a man should be in a position to decide intelligently. The question Dr. Edey raises is whether a man under twenty-five, not yet married, has the experience and/or the foresight to make that intelligent decision. She believes that in most cases he does not. Most authorities agree with her. Still, she recognizes that "there is a body of opinion which says that a person over twenty-one should have the right to decide what to do with his own body."

Dr. Robert B. Benjamin, of Minneapolis's St. Louis Park Medical Center, is part of that "body of opinion." He writes: "All single men requesting vasectomy thus far have been allowed to have the operation. . . . Each request is different. One patient may have frequent relationships with one woman. . . . It would appear, in view of the present sexual revolution, that there will be an increasing number of single men requesting sterilization. To date, all of the single men who have undergone vasectomy have been satisfied. There have been no requests for reversal." [8]

Young *married* men, however, are another story. "I have seen a number of couples," said Dr. Edey, "who have a way of life they enjoy. They both work, they don't want children or they dislike children, and it appears to be a lasting marriage." In such cases, "the odds of the husband changing his mind plummet right down, because he's already found a woman who agrees with him."

A solid marriage is, in fact, essential for a family man considering vasectomy. But some men expect that the vasectomy will work some special magic and cure existing marital ills. It doesn't; on the contrary, it worsens them.

"I recently saw the 'Joneses'—an all too typical example," reports one social worker. "Married because of a pregnancy while still in high school, three children within six years, constant financial and baby care help from both his and her parents, the Joneses had decided on a vasectomy after a difficult third pregnancy. They saw it as the solution to their financial stress and Mrs. Jones's fear of any more pregnancies, which they felt was affecting their sex life.

"But the vasectomy affected their sex life and their marriage even more adversely. It did not help *the real problem,* which was their excessive dependency, impulsiveness, and inability to deal with the normal crises of marriage *in a mature way.*" [9] (Italics added.)

A 1963 study conducted in Iowa showed how devastating a vasectomy can be to marriages already foundering perilously close to the proverbial rocks. This study was somewhat limited, in that it included only twenty-six couples. But it shows what can happen when magical solutions are sought

for difficult problems. "This group," states the report, "saw
the operation [vasectomy] as a 'magical' solution to such
deep-seated problems as 'fear of pregnancy' and sexual
incompatibility." [10] The twenty-six couples, however, were
constantly looking for ready-made answers to complex questions, much the way children do. In fact, the couples' immaturity is apparent throughout the study. The researchers
felt "that this group of couples manifest marked immaturity
in both their courtship patterns and in their marriages, having idealized concepts of marriage as *a way of finding the
satisfactions denied them in their primary families. Many are
'impulse ridden,' given to seeking a simple way out*—a 'magical solution' as it were, of personal problems. . . . *When the
going gets tough in any area, they look for a quick, easy way
out.* Actually, as indicated in the problems manifest before
and after vasectomy, the couples' coping ability seems to
have markedly decreased following the operation. Divorce
or separation then becomes the next simple solution." [11]
(Italics added.)

Admittedly, we are talking about some of life's losers. Of
the twenty-six men in the Iowa study, "eighteen . . . had
a history of acting-out behavior, most frequently described
by the caseworkers as drinking, sexual acting out, irregular
employment, wife beating, gambling, theft, temper tantrums,
financial irresponsibility. Frequently there was a combination of two or more of the above symptoms." [12] And their
wives were not much better. But the point these unfortunate
husbands help illustrate is no less true for other, less troubled
men: vasectomy is not a cure-all, the answer to a maiden's
prayer, the end of all problems. Vasectomy can best be regarded as another ingredient in the total mix of one's life,
including marriage. If the overall mix is a good one, vasec-

tomy will definitely improve it. There is a large body of evidence to support this view.

"Several large follow-up studies among sterilized men have shown that well over 90 percent are pleased with the operation. In a few cases of 'regret' it was found that the men usually had had unrealistic expectations that the operation would resolve such deep-seated sexual problems as impotence or frigidity," [13] reported a recent *New York Times* article. Continually, relentlessly, the data draws us to the same conclusion: men with self-confidence, men who have good feelings about themselves, men who do not feel threatened by other men or by women, men whose love for their wives is more a matter of sharing than it is a matter of dominance —for such men, vasectomy can greatly enhance life.

We have shown that men with sexual problems before the operation do not lose these problems afterward and in fact may intensify them. But what about the man who does not go into the surgeon's office burdened with that psychological load?

"In no instance," reports Dr. Walter R. Stokes, "did a man with a formerly vigorous sex life complain of adverse effects following his vasectomy." [14] Dr. Stokes believes that if a couple are content in their marriage, if they have intelligently and maturely reached a decision about the size of their family, then "a skillfully performed vasectomy is a boon to family life and has no long-range ill effects upon the health or sex performance of the man involved." [15] As a matter of fact, for a great many men, "sex performance" actually improves markedly, as we shall discuss in Chapter 8.

Dr. Henry P. David, Associate Clinical Professor (Psychology) at the University of Maryland Medical School, believes that "a good case can be made that the extent of a

80   *THE TRUTH ABOUT VASECTOMY*

person's ability to master his present and future environment, and govern his own life situation by choosing among socially acceptable alternatives, is a measure of his ego strength and adaptive capacity and thus of his mental health." [16] To which the authors can only add their whole-hearted agreement.

This chapter is entitled "The Machismo Factor" because it deals at some length with the psychological effects of vasectomy on men and masculinity. That is not to suggest that attitudes of women are not of considerable importance, and we shall discuss this in the following chapter. But bear in mind that a very important consideration directly related to the *machismo* factor is sexual performance and enjoyment. We have not ignored it; rather, we believe it important enough to be treated separately.

NOTES

1. Alexander, Bailey: "Vasectomy Is Never Having to Say You're Sorry," *Penthouse Magazine,* November 1971.
2. Ferber, Andrew S., M.D.; Tietze, Christopher, M.D.; Lewit, Sarah: "Men with Vasectomies: A Study of Medical, Sexual and Psychosocial Changes," *Psychosomatic Medicine,* Vol. XXIX, No. 4, July–August 1967.
3. Benjamin, Robert B., M.D.: "Vasectomy as an Office Procedure," *The Bulletin,* St. Louis Park Medical Center, Vol. XIV, No. 1, winter quarter 1970.
4. Ferber, Tietze, and Lewit: *op. cit.*
5. Alexander, Bailey: *op. cit.*
6. Ferber, Tietze, and Lewit: *op. cit.*
7. Edey, Helen M., M.D.: "Psychological Aspects of Vasectomy," *Vasectomy,* "presented by the Center for the Advancement of Population Studies in Medicine and the Student American Medical Association, Ecology Committee," 1972.

8. Benjamin, Robert B., M.D.: *op. cit.*
9. Southwick, Shirley J.: "The Psychological Side Effects of Vasectomy," *The New York Times,* Jan. 14, 1972.
10. Barnes, Elzena, and Johnson, Glenna B.: "Effects of Vasectomy on Marriage Relationships" (A Descriptive Analysis of 26 Cases Seen in Marriage Counseling by Family Service-Travelers Aid, Des Moines, Iowa), 1964.
11. *Ibid.*
12. *Ibid.*
13. Brody, Jane E.: "Sterilization: The Sure Method of Birth Control," *The New York Times,* April 4, 1971.
14. Stokes, Walter R., M.D.: "Long-Range Effects of Male Sterilization," *Sexology,* October 1965.
15. *Ibid.*
16. David, Henry P., Ph.D.: "Mental Health and Family Planning," *Family Planning Perspectives,* Vol. III, No. 2, April 1971.

7

THE WOMAN'S POINT OF VIEW

Among the various causes of sexual problems in women, fear of pregnancy is one of the major ones. The problem worsens if a woman discovers, the hard way, that the various contraceptive methods she has tried do not work for her. An improperly inserted diaphragm, a spermicidal foam or jelly that does not work, inaccurate judgment for the rhythm method, a leaky condom, coitus interruptus that has been ill-timed—all of these have caused "accidental," unwanted pregnancies. The alternatives are an abortion or the responsibility and effort of raising a child, which in many cases is not only a physical and psychological burden but a financial one as well. In some instances an unwanted baby will be given up for adoption. Any one of these choices is at best an extremely difficult decision for a woman to have to make. Well, then, there is always the Pill—unless she has a bad reaction to it. Or forgets to take it.

Of course, a woman can always have herself sterilized—at least, in theory. In practice, however, it is quite another story. The files of the Association for Voluntary Sterilization are filled with court cases throughout the country, instances where women have filed suits against hospitals, doctors, and government authorities because of interference with their "right" to sterilization. Furthermore, female sterilization costs more and is more complicated than male sterilization. (New techniques, however, are constantly being developed. One new method permits a woman to leave the hospital or clinic within hours after she has been sterilized.)

Under such pressures, the sex act, for a woman, can metamorphose from an act of of pleasure and love to one that ranges from indifference to an act of tension, nervousness, and fear. And finally, what was once an expression of mutual love is viewed with revulsion and therefore repulsion. A sexless marriage is a marriage in danger. As a result, according to Dr. David Reuben, "many men turn to vasectomy under pressure from their wives. If a woman tells her husband what's going to happen—or more specifically, what's not going to happen—unless he has his *vas deferens* cut, he really has no choice." [1]

As we have seen in the last chapter, there are some men emotionally unprepared for vasectomy. "If a fellow didn't really want to go through this in the first place," says Dr. Reuben, "but is only pleasing his wife, his emotions can impair his future sexual potency." [2] The FTL Study agrees: ". . . the strongest contraindication for vasectomy is disagreement with one's wife over its advisability." [3]

Such "disagreement with one's wife" is unquestionably a two-sided coin. What if the husband wants to be vasectomized and the wife is against it? It would seem reasonable to ask why a woman would be against her husband's being voluntarily sterilized. The answer, somewhat oversimplified, is that women, just like men, have their prejudices, conflicts, preconceived notions, and unconscious anxieties. These can be manifest in several extremely interesting ways.

A recent article in a professional medical journal dealt with this subject at length. Dr. James A. FitzGerald, an obstetrician-gynecologist whose practice is in upstate New York, discussed women who reacted badly to their husbands' vasectomies. There are two serious flaws in Dr. FitzGerald's paper: first, he gives no statistical data at all; there is no way of discerning whether he is talking about five women or five hundred. Second, he gives no references to other papers or supporting documentation on the same or related subjects. (A professional paper without footnotes is a little like a scrambled egg without salt: digestible, but not very tasty.) Keeping those shortcomings in mind, let us take a look at some of Dr. FritzGerald's findings:

> To some wives, the performance of vas ligation in the male [*sic*] has overtones of willful mutilation. The reasons for the surgery are thought to involve aspects of male, personal selfishness; the results of the surgery may be disturbing because of its irrevocability. Surprisingly, many wives feel that vas ligation makes their husbands more attractive to other women, which does not make a marriage any happier.[4]

A valid concern? Not according to the experts and the studies. "It has been suggested," says Dr. Edey, "that some men seek to be more promiscuous, but in fact follow-up surveys show that an increase in extra-marital affairs after vasectomy is unusual."[5] One of those surveys, the FTL Study, stated: "Only one man reported increased extramarital coitus. He had been having an affair before the vasectomy and was less fearful about it afterward."[6] As a matter of fact, one of the respondents told the investigators: "I think less about other women than I did. I guess it's because I'm more satisfied now." [7]

Apparently keenly attuned to the vagaries of the female mind, Dr. FitzGerald would have us believe that while a woman may be worried about her vasectomized husband chasing around, she is also critical of his performance as a lover. It seems that "their husbands, changed and altered, are frequently subject to a quiet appraisal as lovers. Deficiencies in sexual capabilities which may have existed before vas ligation and which had no reason for recognition are now blamed on the operation. One female complaint is that the sex act 'seems different' or 'less worthwhile.' " [8]

Sexual criticism is only one of the ways in which some women respond negatively to vasectomies. "What happens to these troubled wives is varied. Some of the women's complaints appear somatic in origin; pelvic pain was a common feature of this group, and in addition, elements of metromenorrhagia [uterine bleeding]. Dysmenorrhea [menstrual cramps] often require analgesics." [9]

Adding the information from the preceding chapter to what we have discussed here, the conclusion seems obvious: emotional difficulties, immature marital situations, and a desire for "instant magic" to solve a deep-seated marital problem militate against the husband's vasectomy as much for the wife as they do for him.

Fortunately, those suffering from such adverse psychological effects of male sterilization continue to remain in a tiny minority. "The group I am describing is not numerous," says Dr. FitzGerald, "but it exists. The majority of wives agreeing to male [*sic*] vas ligation accept the alteration in their husbands with relief rather than with an adverse emotional response." [10] Relief seems hardly the word for it.

Many men who undergo vasectomies may be surprised at the seemingly sudden increase in their wives' sexuality. If a man has the emotional stability to undergo a vasectomy, then it is reasonable to assume that he is likely to view such an effect on his wife as an improvement. The result is that everybody is happy. "For many women," says Dr. David Reuben, vasectomy "provides a whole new outlook on sex. For them, it means freedom from the constant low-level anxiety about an 'accident' that could make them a mother again; and they are able to relax and enjoy sexuality with their husbands more than they ever have before.

"Simply because their wives are more responsive, many men find their sexual lives improving as well. As a direct result, their potency may increase dramatically." [11]

Dr. Walter R. Stokes agrees: "I believe that the wives tended to be even more pleased about the results of vasectomy than were the husbands. Many of the wives had become temporarily frigid prior to the operation because of the fear of undesired pregnancy. When they were sure there would be no further pregnancy, they became affectionate with the husband and entered actively into a mutually happy sex life." [12]

Even cold statistics fail to chill the warmth of such reports. The FTL Study shows that "two-thirds of the wives . . . were reported by their husbands as being less tense. . . . Close to four-fifths of the husbands reported that their wives felt less inhibited and freer sexually. . . . Close to two-fifths of the wives were reported by their husbands as initiating love play leading to coitus more often than before the operation. . . ." [13]

All the experts and surveys agree that with the exception of a few women who are likely to have bad reactions to almost anything having to do with sex, vasectomy for a man is a wonderful thing for a woman. The FTL Study sums it up nicely:

> The improvement in the health of the wives . . .
> runs a gamut from decreased premenstrual anxiety,
> through the psychosomatic borderlands of less
> fatigue and lethargy, to improvement in varicose
> veins, all of which seem clearly attributable to not
> being pregnant frequently.[14]

The heightening of sexuality in both the husband and wife after a vasectomy is real, measurable, and translates into increased and improved sexual intercourse, as the next chapter will attempt to demonstrate.

NOTES

1. Reuben, David, M.D.: "Dr. David Reuben Answers Your Questions About Vasectomy," *McCall's,* July 1971.
2. *Ibid.*
3. Ferber, Andrew S., M.D.; Tietze, Christopher, M.D.; Lewit, Sarah: "Men with Vasectomies. A Study of Medical, Sexual and Psychosocial Changes, " *Psychosomatic Medicine,* Vol. XXIX, No. 4, July–August 1967.
4. FitzGerald, James A., M.D.: "The Female Response to Male Vas Ligation," *Medical Insight,* January 1972.
5. Edey, Helen M., M.D.: "Psychological Aspects of Vasectomy," *Vasectomy,* "presented by the Center for the Advancement of Population Studies in Medicine and the Student American Medical Association, Ecology Committee," 1972.
6. Ferber, Tietze, and Lewit: *op. cit.*
7. *Ibid.*
8. FitzGerald: *op. cit.*
9. *Ibid.*

10. *Ibid.*
11. Reuben, David, M.D.: *op. cit.*
12. Stokes, Walter R., M.D.: "Long-Range Effects of Male Sterilization," *Sexology,* October 1965.
13. Ferber, Tietze, and Lewit: *op. cit.*
14. *Ibid.*

8

THE AFTERMATH OF
VASECTOMY

Anyone who has had sexual intercourse more than just a few times is undoubtedly aware that problems and anxieties can seriously interfere with sexual performance and enjoyment. Sometimes the most superficial tensions can affect sexual activity. An argument with the boss, concern over an unpaid bill, depressing news about a relative—anything from a minor annoyance to a major calamity can prevent or disturb sexual pleasure. At some time in his life, every man has probably experienced the frustrating vicious circle in which he finds himself worrying about how he will perform sexually, only to discover that the very fact of worrying prevents him from achieving an erection or causes premature ejaculation.

When such anxieties are temporary and obvious, their impact on sexual activity is also temporary, if not always obvious. But all too often anxieties, particularly those related to sex, are deep-seated, lodged firmly in the unconscious. Thus, an intelligent, well-educated adult can have problems of impotence or frigidity if during childhood he or she was imbued with the concept that sex is dirty, evil, shameful, or sinful. No amount of intellectualizing can dissolve the core of guilt implanted in the unconscious. Similarly, when religion specifically prohibits contraceptive devices, the sex act can become burdened with anxieties if a condom, diaphragm, IUD, or Pill gets into the act.

One of the heaviest emotional burdens an otherwise happy couple often has to bear is concern over yet another pregnancy. Sexual intercourse, constantly advertised as the ultimate expression of love and sharing between a man and a woman, loses some of its glow if, as climax approaches, either the husband or the wife, or both, are silently praying: "God, I hope this doesn't mean another kid!" The fear is well-founded. "It should be emphasized," says Dr. Henry P. David, "that failure rates, even with the most modern, effective contraceptives, still produce a significant number of unwanted births." [1]

The inhibiting aspects of unwanted children could provide enough material for many pages of discussion: the feeling of "encroachment" on the parents' sense of self, the lack of privacy, the "sacrifices" parents are expected to make for children, and so on and on, all worsened by the added burden of guilt many people feel precisely because of their unconscious resentment toward their unplanned children. We dispense with this in only a paragraph here because this is not what this book is about; but these matters are hardly to be glossed over lightly. A father will certainly experience resentment toward both his wife and his children if his wife is too tired at night to have sex with him because "the kids really knocked me out today" or because the house is so crowded that "the kids will hear us." The only small consolation a man may find is in the knowledge that if misery indeed loves company, he has lots of it: this feeling of resentment is as commonplace among fathers as are the baby pictures in their wallets.

While emotional problems and the stresses of anxieties are somewhat intangible, the financial ones are all too apparent. "There's economics: who can afford more children? Ask the man who owns three. Summer camp, orthodontia, guitar lessons, shoes, and all those other tedious necessities are as nothing when arrayed before the humbling $5000 a year required to put Junior through Princeton." [2] Even if Junior should elect to attend a city college or a state university, it costs a great deal of money to keep him alive, fed, clothed, and cared for until the time he is ready to strike out on his own. When a trip to Las Vegas or Paris, many months in the planning, has to be cancelled because a son has managed to crack a couple of ribs during a high school varsity scrimmage, it would take a father with a will of iron and a mother with the soul of a saint to avoid harboring just a little resentment toward the chip off the old block.

It comes as no surprise, therefore, when Dr. Edey tells us, "The number of unplanned children has been somewhat higher in couples choosing vasectomy than the average." [3] Why should a man and woman, otherwise reasonably happy, subject themselves to the pressures of an unwanted pregnancy? If a marriage is relatively stable, it would be foolish to jeopardize that stability when the cause of the problem can be so easily eliminated.

It may be argued that there is always abortion. But this argument contains a built-in absurdity: If the embryo is to be aborted, then the child is unwanted and its conception could have been easily prevented in the first place, accomplishing the same end result. Furthermore, the simple practical facts all favor vasectomy over abortion: sterilization is a one-time proposition, whereas an abortion has to be performed for each unwanted pregnancy; the cost of a vasectomy is almost always lower than the cost of an abortion; and a vasectomy is much easier to obtain than a legal abortion.

Dr. Walter R. Stokes confirms the importance of vasectomy in removing the burden of concern over unplanned children. In discussing candidates for vasectomy, he writes, "Their principal reason in asking for the operation was to stabilize their marriage by closing the door on anxiety over a further pregnancy." [4]

But now another question arises: by "closing the door on anxiety over a further pregnancy," does not one run the risk of opening the door to other anxieties? The Catholic Church believes that the purpose of coitus is reproduction, and that interfering with that purpose is thwarting God's will. To barter the worry over more children for the fear of incurring the wrath of Heaven hardly seems like a sensible exchange. But where there is a will, as the old cliché says, there is a way.

"Some Catholic couples I have talked to," writes Dr. Edey, "prefer voluntary sterilization to contraception because they have sinned once only rather than having to confess to repeated transgression." [5] If Dr. Edey's syntax is a trifle confused, her meaning is not. And the facts seem to bear out Dr. Edey's observation.

In 1963 a study of "330 couples who chose vasectomy as a form of birth control" was conducted by Judson T. Landis, Professor of Family Sociology and a Research Associate at the Institute of Human Development, University of California, Berkeley, and Thomas Poffenberger, who was then Visiting Professor of Child Development at the Baroda (India) University. They found that "although the Catholic

Church is opposed to vasectomy, 19 percent of the men [in the study] and 24 percent of the wives were Catholic." [6] We shall soon see that vasectomy often improves sexual activity, but Landis and Poffenberger reported that "in studying the variables it was found that the greatest change reported in sexual desire was by religion. Of the Catholic men 52 percent reported either strong increase or some increase in sexual desire after the vasectomy in contrast to 35 percent of the Protestant men reporting increased desire." [7] If the theology of having "sinned once only" is arguable, the results, as shown by the statistics, are not.

It would appear that whatever a couple's religious persuasion may be, a vasectomy is generally followed by a sense of well-being. The FTL Study states: "Fifty-three [out of a total of seventy-three couples surveyed] reported an increase in their feelings of over-all happiness, emphasizing such factors as peace, stability, decision-making, and the possibility of planning for the future." [8] It is not difficult to understand the importance of "such factors as . . . planning for the future": one frequently hears couples discuss what they will do "when the children are grown." Such plans do not become practically feasible, however, if there is an unending flow of children, or if the possibility of another pregnancy is always imminent. Frustration is the least serious result in such cases.

Of course, there are some people whose sense of well-being is not improved by vasectomy, but it is likely that in such cases there are other contributing factors. Furthermore, their numbers are almost insignificant when compared with those who feel better after the operation. The Simon Population Trust report states: "A change for the better (579 couples) occurs over a hundred times more frequently than a change for the worse (five couples). Reports of a change for the better (57.3 percent) were appreciably more numerous than reports of no change (42.2 percent). Hence in this sample a majority of the marriages gained in harmony through the husband's vasectomy." [9]

One of the more pleasant ways in which this sense of well-being manifests itself is in increased sexual activity. And why not? If making love is pleasurable, and if vasectomy, as one writer put it, "takes the worry out of being close," then certainly the conditions are right for more frequent love-making. The rate of increase varies greatly from couple to couple, but it is usually discernible to some degree. In the Landis and Poffenberger study, "there was found to be a very wide range in the frequency of intercourse among the respondents. . . . For the entire group the trend was for this frequency to be stepped up after the vasectomy." [10]

Dr. James A. FitzGerald, in his study of women responding adversely to their husbands' vasectomies, stated that the younger the woman, the more likely she was to have a complaint, because, he says, "Age alters sexual performance and tempers interest," [11] a commonly accepted adage. However, if this holds true for the general population, vasectomized men have a different tale to tell. The FTL Study noted "a significant increase in coital frequency at an age when the frequency for the general population is declining." [12] It has been suggested that one of the reasons for the decline of sexual activity in advancing years is fear of pregnancy; a man in his late middle age may not want to become a father. But this is only conjecture; in any case, the fact does remain that vasectomized men do have sex more frequently than their fertile brethren of the same age. Again, as the FTL Study has it: "Although the men were on the average four years older at the time of the interview than they had been at the time of the vasectomy, the mean coital frequency increased from 8.4 to 9.8 times per month, and the median changed from 10.3 to 12.6 times per month. On the basis of data reported by Kinsey and his associates, a decline of 1.2 in mean monthly coital frequency might have been expected in this age interval." [13]

Landis and Poffenberger concur: "Age may be seen as significant here. Our analysis of the age factor showed that it was the men of twenty-five and under at the time of the vasectomy who reported the greatest increase in sexual desire. None of these men reported a decrease in sex desire, and 48 percent reported an increase, while of those who were thirty-eight years old and over, 6 percent reported a decrease in sexual desire and 32 percent reported an increased desire." [14]

It may be argued that sexual frequency is a direct result of the novelty of sterilization. Think of the last time you bought a new car and the number of times, during the first flush of ownership, you took people for a ride around the block. Similarly, a newly vasectomized man is likely to enjoy his new freedom more frequently at first than he will later on, when he gets used to the idea. As Landis and Poffenberger put it: "Another significant difference was observed by how long ago the operation had taken place. Of those who had had the vasectomy more than five years ago 26 percent reported an increase in sex desire while of those who had had the operation less than a year ago 41 percent reported increased sex desire." [15] In other words, while time and age may have a somewhat dampening effect on ardor, the net result is still an overall increase in sexual desire (and, hopefully, in frequency), at least for 26 percent of Landis and Poffenberger's respondents.

Not only are vasectomized men having intercourse more frequently but—and just as important—they and their wives are enjoying it more, another fairly obvious and expected manifestation of the removal of anxiety. The figures may be a trifle dull as statistics, but remember that these represent real people. "Somewhat more than two-thirds of the men (fifty)," says the FTL Study, "stated that they felt freer and less inhibited sexually than before the operation, and somewhat less than one-third (twenty-two) reported no change. . . . According to the men's self-rating of 'over-all satisfaction with coitus' after the operation, three-fourths (fifty-five) were more satisfied, and one-fifth (fifteen) reported no change." [16]

The Simon Population Trust Report not only supports these findings but in the process dispels the myth that the English are cold: "Among men 73 percent and among women over 79 percent report improvement in their sexual lives—nearly three in four men and eight in ten women." [17]

Again, it should be mentioned that not everybody has a better sex life; *many* do. Many do not notice any change one way or the other. And a few actually experience a decline in their sexual activity and/or enjoyment.

The Simon Population Trust Report:

> In respect to *sexual* life, there was no change among a quarter of the men and a fifth of the women, while among the remainder just under fifty times more men and over 150 times more women reported improvements than reported deteriorations. [18]

Landis and Poffenberger:

> The large majority reported that there had been a great increase in enjoyment of the sexual act. Forty-

six percent of the husbands reported that their enjoyment was "much greater" and 49 percent reported that their wives' enjoyment was "much greater"; 24 percent more of the husbands reported enjoyment "somewhat greater" for themselves and 31 percent "somewhat greater" for their wives. . . . Only 2 percent of the husbands reported less enjoyment for their wives.[19]

If you add the "much greaters" to the "somewhat greaters," you will find that a total of 70 percent of the men and 80 percent of the women experienced an increase in enjoyment of the sex act. If there is still a shred of doubt in your mind that anxiety over pregnancy can affect sexual enjoyment, notice, please, that in every case the higher percentages of increased pleasure appear in the women's statistics.

Admittedly, informal, unrecorded studies do not carry quite the clout of well-documented surveys. Nevertheless, it seems worth mentioning that the medical author of this book has performed many hundreds of vasectomies. He cannot recall a single complaint. If there were any, they were probably drowned out by vasectomized men who claim that they now have faster, firmer, and larger erections; that they can sustain the sex act longer; that their wives achieve greater satisfaction from sexual intercourse and have more frequent orgasms; that they (the men) have longer and better orgasms.

And what of those men whose sexual desire and satisfaction diminish after vasectomy? "Three men [of seventy-three studied] stated that they felt less satisfied with their sexual lives after the operation. *Each had a pre-existing potency difficulty* that was aggravated after the operation." [20] (Italics added.)

All may not be lost for such men. If they should change their minds, there is a chance for them to become fathers even though they have become vasectomized. But that chance is a very slim one.

NOTES

1. David, Henry P., Ph.D.: "Mental Health and Family Planning," *Family Planning Perspectives,* Vol. III, No. 2, April 1971.
2. Alexander, Bailey: "Vasectomy Is Never Having to Say You're Sorry," *Penthouse Magazine,* November 1971.
3. Edey, Helen M., M.D.: "Psychological Aspects of Vasectomy," *Vasectomy,* "presented by the Center for the Advancement of Population Studies in Medicine and the Student American Medical Association, Ecology Committee," 1972.
4. Stokes, Walter R., M.D.: "Long-Range Effects of Male Sterilization," *Sexology,* October 1965.
5. Edey, Helen M.: *op. cit.*
6. Landis, Judson T., and Poffenberger, Thomas: "The Marital and Sexual Adjustment of 330 Couples Who Chose Vasectomy as a Form of Birth Control." Paper read before the Research Section of the Annual Meeting of the National Council on Family Relations, Denver, Aug. 23, 1963.
7. *Ibid.*
8. Ferber, Andrew S., M.D.; Tietze, Christopher, M.D.; Lewit, Sarah: "Men with Vasectomies: A Study of Medical, Sexual and Psychosocial Changes," *Psychosomatic Medicine,* Vol. XXIX, No. 4, July–August 1967.
9. "Vasectomy: Follow-up of a Thousand Cases," report by The Simon Population Trust, Cambridge, England, December 1969.
10. Landis and Poffenberger: *op. cit.*
11. FitzGerald, James A., M.D.: "The Female Response to Male Vas Ligation," *Medical Insight,* January 1972.
12. Ferber, Tietze, and Lewit: *op. cit.*
13. *Ibid.*
14. Landis and Poffenberger: *op. cit.*

15. *Ibid.*
16. Ferber, Tietze, and Lewit: *op. cit.*
17. Simon Population Trust: *op. cit.*
18. *Ibid.*
19. Landis and Poffenberger: *op. cit.*
20. Ferber, Tietze, and Lewit: *op. cit.*

9

IF YOU CHANGE YOUR MIND

For a man considering vasectomy, one of the most difficult barriers to cross is the fact that for all practical purposes the operation must be considered irreversible. Despite the optimistic reports, some of which we shall discuss shortly, about the alternatives, a vasectomized man should think of himself as permanently sterile. While sterilization is a 100 percent guarantee of foolproof birth control, the chances of successfully reversing the procedure are considerably lower.

Why should a man want to become fertile again? Some of the answers are obvious: for example, there is the grim but nevertheless very real possibility that some disaster such as an automobile accident could wipe out his entire family. Accident or illness could remove his wife from the scene, and if he should remarry, his second wife might want children of her own. This is also true, of course, in the event of a divorce, especially since in all but the rarest of cases, the children of a broken marriage are placed in the mother's custody. It has been argued that in such instances the man would simply inform his prospective new bride that "biological" children are not possible and if she truly loved him for himself, she would be willing to accept him as he is. Still, if children of her own were part of her overall life plan, she would be unhappy—and therefore, so would he.

While it is true that reasonable and sensible couples consider these possibilities when contemplating sterilization, they tend to dismiss them. "We're willing to take the chance," they claim, usually firm in the belief that "it can't happen to us." In fact, that belief is somewhat justified. While prospects of losing an entire family in one fell swoop certainly exist, they are infinitesimal.

The chances of divorce, however, are considerably greater. In a nation where one out of every three marriages ends up in the matrimonial courts (and there is no telling how many marriages should end up there but don't because of religious, economic, or other reasons), the possibility of a marriage culminating in a divorce should not be taken lightly. However, it should be remembered that the first requirement for seriously considering a vasectomy is a healthy, stable marriage, one in which husband and wife share responsibilities, decisions, desires, ambitions; a marriage in which the lines of communication are open and in constant use. The likelihood of such a marriage dissolving in divorce, with or without vasectomy, is very slim.

Other possible reasons for wanting a reversal of the operation are not so obvious. Remember Dr. Edey's comments about young men who "lack imagination"? A single man in his twenties is very likely to have a considerably different outlook on life from the one he will have when he is thirty-five or forty. It is difficult for most people to accept this likelihood, despite the fact that it is demonstrated to us almost every day of our lives. Do you remember that marvelous piece of furniture you and your wife fell in love with ten years ago? You know, it's the one now moldering in your attic because you can't stand the sight of it and nobody else wants it. Scan the titles of those books you've been hoarding in the storage room or in the uppermost reaches of your bookshelf. How many of them would you like to reread now? If our tastes are capable of changing so dramatically with regard to such relatively trivial matters, how much more likely is the possibility of a change in the desire to have children?

Sometimes a switch is generated by simple economics. It is precisely because some couples love children that they practice birth control. They feel that it is unfair to bring a child into the world unless that child can be provided with adequate medical care, education, and a generally suitable environment, in addition to the simple necessities of food, clothing, and shelter. Such couples will limit the size of their families only to discover, years later, that either because the children have grown and become independent or because the family has improved its station in life, there is more money available and they now want to have more children. Emotions play no small part in such a decision: many couples have children when they are "past their prime" because they miss the kind of animation that leaves a home when children become young adults and strike out on their own.

This is not to suggest that any or all of these possibilities are sufficient to argue against a vasectomy. By far the vast majority of vasectomized men are satisfied with their decision and do not want to undo what has been done. Two physicians, writing in a medical journal, claim that "an estimated 5 percent of vasectomized men may eventually request reversal." [1] This estimate, offered early in 1972, does not coincide with other reports which indicate that less than one percent of vasectomized men seek reversal.

Still, if a vasectomized man should later decide he wants

to become a father, there are three options open to him: (1) surgery; (2) adoption; (3) semen banks. Let's take a close look at each.

Surgery, of course, is usually the method most often considered when the question of reversal comes up. Earlier, we used the term *reanastomosis,* the rejoining of the separated tubes. The procedure itself, when performed on the *vasa deferensa* (plural of *vas deferens*), is called a *vasovasostomy.*

The procedure is almost as simple as the original vasectomy. The surgeon makes an incision in the scrotum, locates the two tied ends of the vas, and reunites them. Dr. Robert B. Benjamin reports that "in very young patients or in others for whom I feel there is a greater likelihood of regretting the procedure, a lesser amount of vas is excised, always in the straight portion, so that the chance of restoration of fertility, should it later be desired, will be about 80 to 90 percent." [2] There are many who would take issue with that figure. Among the confounding mysteries that recur when examining the concept of male sterilization are the wide variations reported in successful reanastomosis, which range from as low as 25 percent to as high as Dr. Benjamin's 80 to 90 percent. The only explanation seems to be that there is some connection between success and the individual surgeon's skills. (But other factors involved have nothing to do with surgical talent, as we shall soon see.)

The passageway in the vas deferens, called the *lumen,* is about as wide as the thickness of a human hair. It is not difficult to appreciate the delicacy required to restore the *patency* (the "openness" and continuity) of the lumen.

Several physicians and other scientists are experimenting with procedures that will circumvent the problem, while at the same time achieving the same effect as vasectomy. If the tube could be blocked in some way without actually severing the vas, then it would be possible to restore fertility at a later time simply by removing the blockage. Extensive research and experimentation are now being conducted with a variety of devices that in some way close off the vas, preventing the flow of sperm through the tube. A tiny incision is made in the vas and a plug is inserted. The vas is then reclosed. The plug may be plastic or metal; some experiments have been tried with silicone. Another method being tried by a distinguished pioneer and researcher is the "Jhaver clip," named for its inventor. Instead of incising the vas, the surgeon places two tiny clips along the duct.

The desired advantage in all these procedures is that should the patient want his fertility restored, a simple surgical procedure removes the *occlusion* (blockage) and eliminates the necessity of attempting to realign the lumen, because it was left undisturbed in the first place.

Perhaps the most sophisticated of all such efforts is a valve on which two prominent scientists are now at work. If successful, this valve would be permanently installed and could be turned on or off virtually at will. The physician, however, would have to do the turning. One can foresee the problems such a device could present if it were possible for its wearer to manipulate it: while it might make social engagements more interesting, the prospects of having the switch moved inadvertently from "off" to "on" could be embarrassing, to say the least.

Do these blocks, plugs, clips, and valves work? Unfortunately, no one knows yet. The experiments are being conducted by conservative and distinguished scientists unwilling to make rash predictions or instill unwarranted optimism. Many of these devices have proved effective in animal experimentation; those that have are now being tested in humans. But the jury is still out. It remains to be seen whether the occluded vas will stretch or expand, so that sperm is permitted to flow around the obstruction. Also, while the substances from which these devices are made are known to be prosthetically safe, there is always the possibility of some as yet unknown side effect resulting from their being placed in the genitals. Also unknown is whether the body will tend to reject artificial devices, as has been known to occur with IUD's.

There is no doubt that in the foreseeable future a simple and safe device that will sterilize men, and will allow for reversibility when desired, will be developed. But even then, it is likely that not all the men so sterilized will become fertile again, for yet another medical mystery arises: even though all systems are restored for the resurgence of sperm, in many men, once the flow is shut off it will not come on again.

Dr. Edey explains that "it has been found that in many men after vasectomy, an apparent antigen-antibody reaction is developed, and even after surgical reanastomosis there may be azospermia [absence of sperm] or the spermatazoa may have a high percent of head-tail separation and are not sufficiently viable to cause pregnancy. This phenomenon will be a problem with any of the supposedly reversible techniques which are under study or being proposed, such as plugs, clips, or intra-vas devices, and the operation must be considered irreversible at this time." [3]

An *antigen* is a chemical that the body produces to manufacture antibodies. An *antibody* is another substance that the body produces to protect against other "bodies." It is the antibodies in your system that fight off bacteria and make it possible for you to survive the common cold or to resist serious infection when you nick yourself shaving. Although no one knows exactly how or why, the body apparently produces an antibody that acts against sperm which have been absorbed into the bloodstream after vasectomy. Certainly this is not a cause for concern. The vasectomized man is completely unaware that this is happening, and there are absolutely no adverse effects on his general health or on his sense of well-being. All it means is that the body has geared itself to react against sperm and once having done so, will not wind down, even after a surgically successful reanastomosis.

According to Drs. Richard D. Amelar and Lawrence Dubin, "Provided the occluding operation has been performed in the straight portion of the vas, well away from the convolutions adjacent to the epididymis, a skilled urologist should be able to accomplish successful reanastomosis about 70 percent of the time, with reappearance of sperm cells in the ejaculate. But only 25 percent of reoperated men will be able to impregnate their wives. The failures may be caused by sperm-agglutinating and sperm-immobilizing antibodies. In 1971, Dr. R. Ansbacher reported finding these in 54 percent of patients six months after vasectomy." [4] *Agglutinating* means "sticking together." Whether the sperm cells are "glued" to each other or "immobilized," the end result is the same.

Even if these antibodies do not appear, it is still possible to have a surgically successful reanastomosis that is a functional failure. When sperm leave the epididymis and enter the vas, they are helped along the way by a system of sympathetic nerves. Apparently, a nervous system that has been rendered unnecessary by vasectomy stops functioning. "It is also possible," say Amelar and Dubin, "the vas ligation may interrupt the sympathetic nervous system control of the vas' spontaneous motility. This would interfere with sperm transport mechanisms even after vas reanastomosis." [5]

Matthew Freund, Ph.D., is Professor of Pharmacology

and Associate Professor of Obstetrics and Gynecology at New York Medical College. He has studied this interesting phenomenon and concluded that "the question, will this sympathetic nerve supply regenerate after vasovasostomy, remains unanswered. Without an intact sympathetic nerve supply to the proximal [connected] vas and to the epididymis, it is difficult to see how complete recovery in sperm output after vasovasostomy . . . can be achieved." Dr. Freund, with the conservatism of the careful scientist, sums up matters neatly: "The results of vasovasostomy have not been good and workers in this field do not yet fully understand the reasons for the lack of success in surgical restoration." [6]

Put briefly, for a vasovasotomy to be effective, three conditions must prevail: the reanastomosis must be perfect; there must be no antibodies that affect the sperm; the sympathetic nervous system of the vas must be intact and in working order. An average estimate is that 25 percent of all men seeking reversal of their vasectomies will become fertile again. Continued and increased research may be able to raise that figure some day. But there is no doubt that part of the "problem" is that there are so few men on whom the necessary tests can be performed, because so few men who have been vasectomized *want* to become fertile again.

As has been previously pointed out, only about 3 percent of all vasectomized men have any regrets, and those regrets invariably stem not from sterility but from injury to their faith in magic: they expected the vasectomy to be an instant cure for marital ills. These men are not likely to submit their genitalia to yet another operation like a vasovasostomy. The fact that so few men are available to enable proper research into reversal of vasectomy is undoubtedly one of the highest tributes to voluntary sterilization.

Adoption is another option if a vasectomized man decides he wants to become a father. It is usually regarded as an example of man's better nature. Unwed mothers who give their babies up for adoption can ease the pain of losing the child with the knowledge that the infant will be loved and properly cared for. Ecologists are all in favor of adoption because it allows people to have children without adding to the already perilously swollen population. Adoptive parents feel justifiably proud because they have rescued a tiny human being from the dreariness of an institutionalized life and they are giving the child love, warmth, understanding, care—in short, a good home.

But even under the most ideal conditions, adoption has never been easy. Efforts to match a baby with prospective parents are not always successful, especially when such factors as religious background enter into the picture. Thus, for example, because of the few babies put up for adoption by Jewish mothers, Jewish couples have always had difficulty adopting and have often met with failure. Another obstacle to be contended with is the adoption agency's approval of the prospective parents. The agency will carefully consider the home environment; economic, social, and educational status; the ages; and the general psychological condition of the applicants.

In recent years, babies available for adoption have become even more scarce, making the procedure still more difficult. Paradoxically, those couples best able to adopt children— from an economic and educational point of view—are least likely to get them, because the liberalized abortion laws have practically removed Caucasian babies from the adoption market. It is the white, middle-class American couple who are most likely to be interested in adoption and best able to afford it, but it is also the white middle-class mother-to-be who is most likely to consider abortion and is best able to afford it.

Of course, there is no logical reason why a white couple cannot adopt a black, Asian, Indian, or other nonwhite child. But as we have said so often, logic and emotions are two different things.

The whole subject of adoption is an extremely complex one and deserves treatment as a separate study. For our purposes, it will suffice to say that as a possible means of "reversing" the effects of vasectomy, adoption can be a difficult and often unattainable alternative.

A number of vasectomy candidates are taking advantage of a relatively recent innovation: the human semen bank. Although the various facilities that are available have somewhat different approaches to the concepts of sales and promotion of their services, their methods of operation are essentially the same. The "depositor" visits the laboratory several weeks prior to his scheduled vasectomy, bringing with him a fresh specimen of his semen. (Semen can also be produced on the premises, in a small, private room provided for that purpose.) After the semen is tested for the sperm's quantity, condition, and motility, the specimen is divided into a number of little tubes, usually about thirty-six, and placed in liquid nitrogen, which has a temperature of 321° below zero. At any time in the future, upon request from a physician, the frozen semen is removed, thawed, and the physician uses the tube as part of a special syringe with which to inseminate the prospective mother.

Idant Corporation and Genetic Laboratories, Inc., the two most publicized semen banks, both agree to store the semen for a period of ten years. But there is a bit of controversy surrounding the ten-year limit. The American Public Health Association advised the readers of its publication, *The Na-*

tion's Health: "Findings of Edward T. Tyler, M.D., of Los Angeles, a specialist in artificial insemination, show that children have been born to mothers impregnated with sperm frozen up to two-and-a-half years. Other researchers, such as Emil Steinberger, M.D., University of Texas School of Medicine, have made more conservative estimates, citing sixteen months as the longest documented time period in which sperm has been frozen, thawed, and then used successfully to impregnate a woman." [7] Dr. Jerome Silbert, Idant's Director of Laboratories, told the authors that human semen has been shown to be fertile after ten years of freezing, but in the APHA article quoted above, it was reported that "Silbert said his consultant, Dr. J. K. Sherman, a biologist, has reported ten years as the longest successful freezing period, although, Silbert acknowledged, the report is 'not in the literature.' " [8] (Note: the article appeared in February 1972.)

The fact that distinguished scientists are affiliated with both firms has not alleviated some of the trepidation that exists. *Medical World News* commented: "One big problem that worries authorities in the field . . . is that there are very few laws controlling sperm banks. And considering the profits the operators of such banks might be able to reap, the temptation for them to oversell customers on the possibility of success could be considerable." [9] It would appear that so far, none of the banks has succumbed to that temptation. The literature disseminated by Idant and Genetic Laboratories offers no more that a 60 to 70 percent probability of successful pregnancy from frozen semen, and it seems to us that the relatively low cost is worth the gamble. There is an initial fee of about eighty dollars, followed by a yearly maintenance fee averaging eighteen dollars. (These figures may vary slightly from one bank to another and may depend on possible variations in laboratory procedure as determined by the composition and nature of the semen.) Should a "depositor" fail to maintain his payments, the abandoned semen is used for research and experimentation, but *never* for artificial insemination. (See Appendix C for a list of semen banks.)

Should a man decide to undergo a vasectomy, he should be aware that through vasovasostomy, adoption, or artificial insemination, he may still be able, at some future date, to father children. But he must also understand that in all probability, voluntary sterilization means permanent sterilization. He must reconcile himself to the likelihood that once a vasectomy is performed, he will be forever sterile. For some men, that likelihood spells calamity. For millions of others, it spells emancipation.

In which category do you belong?

NOTES

1. Amelar, Richard D., M.D., and Dubin, Lawrence M.D.: "Vasectomy: An Increasingly Popular Alternative," *Medical World News,* March 3, 1972.
2. Benjamin, Robert B., M.D.: "Vasectomy as an Office Procedure," *The Bulletin,* St. Louis Park Medical Center, Vol. XIV, No. 1, winter quarter 1970.
3. Edey, Helen M., M.D.: "Sterilization," *New York Medicine,* August 1970.
4. Amelar and Dubin: *op. cit.*
5. *Ibid.*
6. Freund, Matthew, Ph.D.: "Reversibility of Vasectomy and the Role of the Frozen Semen Bank," *Medical Counterpoint,* Vol. III, No. 11, November 1971.
7. "Population Council Cautions Men Not to Depend on Frozen Sperm," *The Nation's Health,* February 1972.

8. *Ibid.*
9. "Frozen Sperm: Word of Warning," *Medical World News,* March 3, 1972.

10

IS VASECTOMY FOR YOU?

Michael Newman is an intelligent, well-paid office manager who married a divorcée with two children. At the time of his marriage he was thirty-nine, his wife thirty-four. Two years later, they had a son; a year after that, another son was born. Shortly after the birth of the second child, one of the authors suggested to Michael that perhaps he would now consider sterilization. It was understandable that in addition to the family Michael acquired upon his marriage, he would want natural children of his own, but now that he had two, why not heed the advice of ecologists and help to maintain a controlled population. Michael's response was one of heated indignation.

"My wife and I happen to be two highly intelligent people," he declared. "Why should we limit our family? We're doing the world a favor by populating it with intelligent children. If you want to preach population control, start with those chiselers on welfare who keep having more and more children just so they can collect fatter checks."

It would have been pointless to attempt to convince this man that population control is everybody's responsibility, that concerted efforts are being made to educate *all* segments of the population about the menace of a high birth rate, but that it is easier to begin with those who are already educated, especially the highly intelligent. Michael's response was based not on reason but on his personal needs, ambitions, and values . . . not to mention a modicum of bigotry.

Several months later, quite suddenly and surprisingly, Michael raised the subject again: "By the way, how much does a vasectomy cost?" When asked what made him reconsider, he replied: "Well, I figured out that on an office manager's salary, no matter how high I might go, a wife, four kids, and a mortgage are about all I'll ever be able to handle." And what about population control? Did the very real prospects of worldwide famine, bloody battles for land space, widespread unemployment, high percentages of pollution, a rapid decline in human values compensated for by an equally rapid increase in crime and violence—did none of these things affect his decision to limit the size of his family? "Don't be ridiculous," he snapped. "What's that got to do with anything?"

Before you condemn Michael for his apparent selfishness, think how you would react in a similar situation. You have probably noticed that this is the first time we have seriously raised the subjects of population control and ecology. It is not that we are not concerned about it; we are. We could, as others have done, cite figures on population and poverty from India to Brazil. We could prove, with copious documentation, that unless drastic and dramatic steps are taken immediately, in twenty or thirty years there will not be sufficient air fit to breathe, that pure water will become nonexistent, that food supplies and energy sources will be sapped within our children's lifetimes.

We desperately wish we could convince every man in the

world to limit the size of his family to two children, and we could back up that plea with some very convincing arguments. You would listen, shake your head sadly, and agree: they really ought to do something about it. "They," not you. Because when it gets down to cases, the average man does not think about things like ecology and population control when he considers placing himself in the hands of a surgeon. He thinks about himself, his wife, his family, his own lifestyle. We neither condemn nor condone this attitude; we merely recognize it for the truth that it is. There are some men who are concerned with the fate of the human race and undergo vasectomies out of a sense of responsibility to mankind. Such men are rare, and even they do not become sterile without first considering the consequences of such an act on their own lives. This is as it should be, for no man can be of any value to others unless he is of value to himself. Therefore, when you consider whether vasectomy is for you, we hope you will keep in mind that you have a responsibility to the human race. But we also hope you will always remember that your first responsibility is to yourself and to your family.

We now offer you an opportunity that many people secretly crave but rarely achieve: a chance to play God. Here are five actual case studies of men who have come to a surgeon or a clinic requesting vasectomy. You decide which, if any, should have their request granted. (All names, of course, are fictitious.)

CASE NO. 1. Bill Arnold, thirty-nine, and his wife Helen, thirty-six, have been married for seventeen years. They have five children, ranging from sixteen to three. Bill works as a truckdriver's assistant; with overtime and some occasional moonlighting he averages about $12,000 a year.

The Arnolds are Catholics, but only Helen and the children go to confession and attend church. Helen would like Bill to be more observant, but she is not concerned about it. She feels it is a matter between Bill and his conscience.

In recent years, Bill and Helen's sex life has not been very exciting. Bill is concerned about still another child and Helen does not like to use contraception—although again, as long as Bill uses condoms, she feels it is not her responsibility or her sin. She could never use a diaphragm or take the Pill, however.

Should Bill Arnold be vasectomized?

CASE NO. 2. Frank Pearson, twenty-eight, is product manager for a large manufacturer of cosmetics. He is in line for a vice-presidency, and already "headhunters" from rival companies are dangling tempting salaries before him. He will be earning over thirty thousand dollars a year before he is thirty years old. His wife, Nancy, twenty-five, is a buyer in a medium-size department store, with an annual salary of seventeen thousand dollars.

The Pearsons, both college graduates, have been married for three years. When Frank proposed to Nancy, he told her that he was very ambitious, intended to make a great deal of money as quickly as possible, and then enjoy what he made by traveling and living well. He was not particularly interested in children because they would probably interfere with his long-range plans. He did, however, want Nancy to share his life with him. That was fine with her, as long as she would be permitted to pursue her own career.

Nancy had grown up in an atmosphere dominated by adults and had never felt very comfortable around children. She was perfectly satisfied with the idea of a husband who would not demand that she present him with an heir.

Frank and Nancy agreed that if a child should come along —by accident—there would be no difficulty in coping with it. Except for the brief period of confinement, Nancy would be free to continue working because in addition to the other luxuries their combined incomes permitted, they could certainly afford a governess. Nancy is on the Pill and has some trepidation about prolonged exposure to it. Neither Frank nor Nancy trust other forms of contraception.

Frank Pearson wants a vasectomy; his wife approves wholeheartedly. Should he have one?

CASE NO. 3. Alex Fine has been married and divorced twice. His first wife has remarried, and her husband has legally adopted Alex's two children, so Alex no longer has to pay her alimony or child support.

His second wife works and does not demand alimony, insisting only that Alex pay for the support of their one child, which he can easily manage from the comfortable income derived from his hardware store. Alex sees his children occasionally, but the meetings are always strained and awkward.

Now, at forty-five, Alex does not want to live alone anymore. He would like to remarry, and there are several women who would probably have him. But he doesn't want to be talked into fathering any more children. After his vasectomy, he would propose to his first choice and explain that he is sterile. If that did not suit her, well, he would simply have to find someone else. Children at his age would be a headache. Besides, having tried marriage twice and failed, there was certainly no assurance he would make a go of it the third time. Why risk the burden of yet another bite out of his income for child support?

Alex Fine is convinced that the best thing for him is a vasectomy. Is he right?

CASE NO. 4. Al Parris describes himself as "a lover of the old school." He likes his sex hot, heavy, and often, as indicated by the fact that at the age of twenty-five, he is the father of three children, with another on the way. Marie, twenty-three, married Al six years ago, when she was still in high school and already pregnant with their first child.

Marie has tried the Pill and reacted very badly to it. Al finds a diaphragm aesthetically offensive, so they rely on condoms, which in the heat of passion he sometimes forgets to use. Marie has become increasingly reluctant to have sex, and Al resents her seeming lack of participation in intercourse; he considers it a reflection on him.

Four or five times since their marriage, Al has had extramarital sex. These were always very casual and brief relationships. Al rationalizes that when Marie turns her back on him, he has to prove to himself that he is a real man, so if he "fools around a little," it is really her fault.

Al's impulses do not stop in the bedroom. He cannot resist temptation, and although his extravagances are often manifested in presents for Marie and the children, he is nevertheless heavily in debt. Al is a skilled carpenter but he doesn't like working for others, so he hires himself out as an independent contractor. Unfortunately, work is not too plentiful, and in a good year he can count on nine to ten thousand dollars.

Al Parris is frustrated by his wife's lack of interest in sex. He is convinced that if he has a vasectomy, and "takes the worry out of being close," Marie will love him again and their tense, nearly incendiary home life will be replaced by the torrid sex they shared in the early days of their marriage.

If you were Al's doctor, would you perform a vasectomy?

CASE NO. 5. Walter Farrell became a police officer when he was twenty-one years of age. Now a sergeant, he is looking forward to his retirement in four years, when he will be forty-six and will have served twenty-five years on the force. He will receive half his sergeant's salary for the rest of his life. That, plus his pension fund, some judicious investments, and savings, should see him through for the rest of his days. Walter and Lucille have two children, a boy eighteen and a girl sixteen. Walter Jr. has just entered college, and Sally will follow him in two years. The money for their education has already been set aside.

Lucille Farrell, thirty-nine, is secretly pleased that her husband still finds her attractive and desirable after twenty years of marriage. She and Walter enjoy an active, vigorous sex life. Lucille has been on the Pill for about six years, on and off, believing that it is better not to take it continuously. When she is not using the Pill, she uses a diaphragm. The Farrells love children and they are looking forward to grand-children, but they do not want any more babies of their own.

They have considered vasectomy and have asked their physician for his advice. What would you advise?

Now that our little game is over, we must confess that we have not played fairly. The fact is that whatever answers you gave are correct. It might have helped a little if, at the outset, we had insisted that you be objective. But that is precisely the point: it is almost impossible to be objective about steri-lization, and because your answers were probably based on your own values and influenced by your own circumstances, the answers you gave, whatever they are, were right—for you.

The right answers for us are four yeses and one no. In our opinion, Al Parris, No. 4, should not be vasectomized. From the scant information given, it would seem that Al is imma-ture and irresponsible. He is unwilling to share the burden of his growing family, shunting the blame to his wife and to his "natural drives" as "a lover of the old school." He ex-pects vasectomy to set everything right again, but he is wrong. When he finds that his wife is still cool toward him, that his financial situation is no more secure, that his children still make demands on him, he may well regret his vasectomy. What Al needs is not sterilization but a good marriage counselor at the very least. A little psychiatric help might go a long way with Al Parris.

But what about you? Chances are that none of the five cases exactly matches your own circumstances. Whether or not you should have a vasectomy is a decision only you can make, together with your wife and your physician. But we can offer some guidelines. Your decision should be based in large part upon your answers to the following ten questions:

1. Are you in good physical health? Do not even contemplate surgery of any kind if you are not well (unless, of course, there is some emergency). If you are cheating on that annual physical checkup that you know you ought to have, now is the time to make up for your lapse. Get checked out by a doctor before you even consider a vasectomy.

2. Are you in good mental health? If you are presently under any kind of stress, anxiety, or tension, it might be better to forget about sterilization for the time being. A vasectomy is an important step and, as we have explained, an irrevocable one. Your mind should be free from care so that you can make your decision intelligently.

If there are pressures on the job, if there are problems at home, or if there is some persistent problem disturbing your peace of mind, take care of those problems first.

On the other hand, if the stress, anxiety, or tension derives from concern over an unwanted pregnancy, then a vasectomy is probably the best way to restore your peace of mind.

3. Do you have confidence in your own manhood? There are many men who believe that the criterion for manhood rests in the groin. The size of such a man's masculinity is measured by the length of his erect penis. Al Parris, in Case No. 4, is a perfect example. Al does not want any more children, but unconsciously he associates the ability to make babies with his qualifications as a man. If that ability were to be removed, part of his manhood would go with it.

There are, however, many more men who measure manhood by more valid criteria: a capacity for love; a desire to provide the best they can for their wives and children; an ambition to do their work well; an appreciation of the needs and feelings of those around them. These criteria have nothing to do with fertility. In fact, a man's reliance on them can often be demonstrated by his having a vasectomy. In many cases, this is one way of showing that he really cares about his wife and children.

4. Do you have confidence in your own sexuality? Being fertile and being "sexy" are not the same thing. If you believe that they are, then in the final analysis, sex for you is really a device for baby-making and nothing more.

We do not happen to agree with you. We believe that sex is an expression of and an outgrowth of love, that it is the most perfect way for a man and woman to share each other, and that not incidentally it is a lot of fun. If you disagree, then you should think twice about being vasectomized.

If, however, you share our point of view, then it will be apparent to you that you can be as sexual after vasectomy as before. Many men, in fact, become even "sexier" because the baby-making factor has been removed and there is no anxiety to impede the pleasure of the act of love.

5. *Does your wife fully understand what a vasectomy involves?* This is a complicated and extremely important question. Certainly, with the use of a simple diagram like the one in this book, it is no problem to explain to your wife how a vasectomy is performed and what it accomplishes. But this question goes well beyond that. Your wife must know more than the mere physiology of vasectomy; she must be fully aware of what it will mean to you, what it will mean to her, and what it will mean to your life together. Unless you and your wife communicate with each other, think twice before you become sterilized.

Most husbands and wives snicker with contempt when it is suggested that they do not communicate. Yet, we constantly read or hear of couples who sue for divorce after ten, fifteen, even twenty years of marriage. The reasons are varied and complex, but they often boil down to this: after twenty years of working hard, raising children, and building a home, the husband and wife finally have an opportunity to relax, to spend time with each other, to talk to each other. To their dismay, they discover that they have nothing to say. Unfortunately, it is usually because the husband, "out there in the world," has outgrown his wife intellectually. Hopefully, this is changing, but there are still wide gaps in communication between husband and wife.

Charles and Edith Hanley, a happily married couple by any standard, unwittingly offered the authors astonishing proof of how a lack of communication can exist between people who have lived together for over twenty years. Charles was privately interviewed at length as part of the research for this book. He is absolutely dead set against vasectomy, and in an effort to discover a little more about the "machismo factor," we wanted to know why. For all practical purposes, the question is academic: Charles, fifty-two, has two sons and a daughter, all nearly adult, and he does not want any more children. Still, he is opposed to sterilization because he feels that the inability to impregnate a woman "takes something out of the sex act."

How, we asked, does Edith feel about it? "Oh," he replied, "I don't think it matters to her one way or the other. She doesn't want any more children, either—she's forty-three, you know—and she couldn't care less about my fertility."

Later, in another private interview, we questioned Edith. How would she feel if Charles had a vasectomy? "Terrible," she said, "just awful!"

Why? Would she like to become pregnant again?

"Well," she admitted, "I wouldn't mind. I'm not planning on it, mind you, but if an accident should happen, I'd be very happy about it."

And what if Charles were to become sterile as the result of an accident or as a precautionary measure following a prostatectomy? Would that make Charles less of a man in Edith's eyes?

"In all honesty," she said, "I'm afraid it would. I know all the arguments. He would still be the same wonderful husband he's been all these years. We don't plan to have any more children, anyway. What difference could it possibly make? The answer is I don't know. I just know it wouldn't be the same."

Fortunately, most women do not share Edith's views, but the fact remains that Charles is totally unaware of how his wife feels about the subject of vasectomy. He thinks she is indifferent about it. Edith is totally unaware of Charles' misconception of her feeling and unless one has in the meantime told the other, the situation still exists. It is only by a stroke of luck that the end result of their different views comes out the same: they are both opposed to the idea of vasectomies.

But that does not change the fact that a serious lack of communication exists between a happily married couple.

6. Do you have a stable marriage? This is a question only you and your wife can answer, for what may seem like a stable marriage to you could be viewed as a dull, humdrum existence by some, or as a life full of hedonistic orgies by others. If you or your wife see sterilization as a cure for marital ills, chances are the trouble lies elsewhere.

In a strong, stable marriage, a vasectomy is seen as a positive step forward, one that further stabilizes an already good relationship.

7. Are you certain about the size of your family? We hope you will decide to limit your family to two children or, if you already have more than two, that you will stop now. But you and your wife must examine the question carefully. Some couples, especially when they are young, are convinced that children would stand in the way of their careers or impede the life-style they are carving out for themselves. But they may change their minds once they have achieved their goals. Others are experiencing economic pressures and feel that more children would only add to an already weighty burden. Once that burden is removed, they may regret their decision.

If you find yourself saying: "Sure, I'd like more kids—if I could afford them," then you must consider the possibility that some day you *will* be able to afford them. If, on the other hand, you are saying: "Things are just fine the way they are right now, and I want them to stay that way," then you are probably a good candidate for vasectomy.

8. If you are unmarried, or if, by accident or choice, you should become single again, are you prepared to face the fact that you will not father any children? Being sterile is no great calamity. As Dr. Edey often points out, many men discover that they are sterile because of some accident, illness, or biological malfunction. They are the same men the day after they find out as they were the day before they found out. The point to remember is that vasectomy is not a gamble; you are not taking a chance. It is an irreversible certainty.

9. Are you free of any guilt or recriminations? Someone once said that there are no atheists in foxholes. That bit of folksy philosophy simply means that no matter how sophisticated, blasé, or cynical we may become, there is always the probability that when caught in a bind, our earliest training and indoctrination come to the fore.

If you have ever been taught that sex without reproduction is morally wrong or religiously sinful, then you must be certain, beyond a shadow of a doubt, that you no longer believe it. Or, as many have done, you may be able to reconcile yourself to the belief that while sex without offspring is bad, bringing unwanted children into the world is worse.

A startling observation was offered the authors by a man who had studied for a decade to become a Jesuit priest: "I left the order a year before my ordination because I finally realized that the Church's position on birth control was immoral." This viewpoint is perhaps a bit strong, but it is at least an honest one.

Examine your own conscience and your own beliefs. Vasectomy is irreversible and you must live with your decision for the rest of your life.

10. Do you fully understand what a vasectomy is and is not? Simply stated, a vasectomy is a simple operation that usually has no adverse physical effects and causes no changes except to make a man permanently sterile. But you now know that there is much more to it than that. It can have a profound and important effect on your entire life, and on your family's.

If you have answered "Yes" to each of these ten questions, then we believe that effect will be a good one. We believe your life will be happier, more fulfilling, more rewarding. Your sex life will be better because you and your wife will enjoy it more. You and she will have peace of mind and will be drawn even closer together. Obviously, we are in favor of vasectomy when conditions are right.

Only you can decide if they are.

APPENDIX A
SAMPLE
VASECTOMY RELEASE FORM

CONSENT FOR STERILIZATION

(Date)   , 19

We hereby consent to the performance of a sterilizing operation on _____
by Dr._____, and release him and any participating in the operation from all claims either of us might have because of the operation.

We are of age, are mentally competent, and understand that the operation is intended to prevent pregnancy.

Witness: _____
                                              (Wife)

_____   _____
                                           (Husband)

_____   _____
                                           (Address)

Prepared with legal advice by

Association for Voluntary Sterilization
14 W. 40th St.
New York, N.Y. 10018

APPENDIX B
VASECTOMY CLINICS
(AND HOSPITALS IN WHICH VASECTOMY IS PERFORMED AS AN OUTPATIENT PROCEDURE)

The following list was supplied through the courtesy of the Association for Voluntary Sterilization, Inc. The names of the various facilities were obtained from diverse sources by AVS, and sometimes there is conflicting information about the program of a particular facility. The prudent vasectomy candidate would be wise, therefore, to check out the facility by letter or telephone before visiting.

An asterisk (*) indicates those facilities reported as performing vasectomy as an outpatient procedure.

ALABAMA

Planned Parenthood of
   Birmingham Area, Inc.
1714 11th Avenue South
Birmingham 35205

ALASKA

*Anchorage Community
   Hospital
825 L Street
Anchorage 99501

ARIZONA

Planned Parenthood
   Association of Phoenix
1200 South Fifth Avenue
Phoenix 85003

Pima County Health
   Department
Pima County General
   Hospital
2900 South Sixth Avenue
Tucson 85713

Planned Parenthood of
Tucson
127 South Fifth Avenue
Tucson 85701

*Tucson Medical Center
Grant Road at Beverly
Tucson 85712

CALIFORNIA

*Delta Memorial Hospital
3901 Lone Tree Way,
Box 236
Antioch 94509

*Alta Bates Community
Hospital
Webster at Regent
Berkeley 94705

*Herrick Hospital
2001 Dwight Way
Berkeley 94704

*American River Health Care
Center
4747 Engle Road
Carmichael 95608

*Eden Hospital
20103 Lake Chabot Road
Castro Valley 94546

*Laurel Grove Hospital
19933 Lake Chabot Road
Castro Valley 94546

*Concord Community
Hospital
2540 East Street
Concord 94520

*Fresno Community Hospital
Fresno and R Streets
Fresno 93720

*Glendale Adventist Hospital
1504 East Wilson Street
Glendale 91206

Planned Parenthood of
Hayward
1252 B Street
Hayward, 94541

*Scripps Memorial Hospital
9888 Genessee Avenue
Box 28
La Jolla 92037

Loma Linda Medical Center
Vasectomy Service
11234 Anderson Street
Loma Linda 92354

*Memorial Hospital Medical
Center of Long Beach
2801 Atlantic Avenue
Long Beach 90806

Planned Parenthood–World
Population
3100 West 8th Street
Los Angeles 90005

UCLA Medical Center
10833 Le Conte Avenue
Los Angeles 90024

*White Memorial Medical
Center
1700 Brooklyn Avenue
Los Angeles 90033

Women's Hospital Vasectomy
Clinic
USC Medical Center
1200 North State Street
Los Angeles 90033

Contra Costa County
Medical Services
(Outpatient clinics in
Richmond and Pittsburg)
2500 Alhambra Avenue
Martinez 94553

*El Camino Hospital
2500 Grant Road
Mountain View 94040

*Hoag Memorial
Hospital–Presbyterian
301 Newport Boulevard
Newport Beach 92660

*Highland General Hospital
1411 East 31st Street
Oakland 94602

Birth Control Institute, Inc.
1818 West Chapman Avenue
Orange 92668

*Orange County Medical
Center
101 South Manchester
Avenue
Orange 92668

Orange County Planned
Parenthood
704 North Glassell
Orange 92667

*Stanford University Hospital
300 Pasteur Drive
Palo Alto 94304

*South California Permanente
Medical Group
13652 Cantara Street
Panorama City 91402

*Pittsburg Community
Hospital
550 School Street
Pittsburg 94565

*Parkview Community
Hospital
3865 Jackson Avenue
Riverside 92503

*Riverside General Hospital
9851 Magnolia Avenue
Riverside 92503

*Sacramento Medical Center
2315 Stockton Boulevard
Sacramento 95817

*Sutter Memorial Hospital
52nd and F Streets
Sacramento 95819

San Bernardino County
Health Department
315 Mountain View Avenue
San Bernardino 92401

Planned Parenthood of San
Diego County
1172 Morena Boulevard
San Diego 92110

Cathedral Hill Medical
Center
1801 Bush Street
San Francisco 94109

*Permanente Medical Group
2200 O'Farrell Street
San Francisco 94115

Planned Parenthood–World
Population Center
Vasectomy Clinic
2340 Clay Street
San Francisco 94115

*San Francisco General
1001 Potrero Avenue
San Francisco 94110

*University of California
    Hospitals and Clinics
San Francisco 94122

Family Planning Alternatives
265 Meridian Avenue
San Jose 95126

Harold D. Chope
    Community Hospital
222 West 39th Avenue
San Mateo 94403

San Mateo Planned
    Parenthood Vas Clinic
373 South Claremont
San Mateo 94401

*Brookside Hospital
Vale Road
San Pablo 94806

*Marin General Hospital
250 Bon Air Road, Box 2129
San Rafael 94901

Santa Barbara Planned
    Parenthood
400 Laguna Street
Santa Barbara 93101

Moore–Liebel Medical
    Corporation
7 West 5th Street
Stockton 95206

*Harbor General Hospital
1000 West Carson Street
Torrance 90502

Solano County Health
    Department Vasectomy
    Clinic
228 Broadway
Vallejo 94591

*Kaiser Foundation Hospital
1425 South Main Street
Walnut Creek 94596

COLORADO

*Memorial Hospital
1400 East Boulder Street
Colorado Springs 80909

Denver General Hospital Vas
    Clinic
West Sixth Avenue and
    Cherokee Street
Denver 80204

Eitzsimmon's General
    Hospital
Peoria and East Colfax
    Streets
Denver 80240

Rocky Mountain Planned
    Parenthood
2025 York Street
Denver 80205

CONNECTICUT

*Hartford Hospital
80 Seymour Street
Hartford 06115

*Mt. Sinai Hospital
500 Blue Hills Avenue
Hartford 06112

Planned Parenthood League
    of Connecticut
406 Orange Street
New Haven 06511

DELAWARE

*Wilmington Medical Center
Box 1668
Wilmington 19899

DISTRICT OF COLUMBIA

*Freedman's Hospital
6th and Bryant Street, N.W.
Washington, D.C. 20001

*George Washington
University Hospital
901 23rd Street, N.W.
Washington, D.C. 20031

Pre-Birth Clinic
1028 Connecticut Avenue,
N.W.
Washington, D.C. 20006

PRETERM Vasectomy
Clinic
1726 I Street, N.W.
Washington, D.C. 20006

*Washington Hospital Center
110 Irving Street, N.W.
Washington, D.C. 20010

FLORIDA

*Broward General Medical
Center
1600 South Andrews Avenue
Fort Lauderdale 33316

*Memorial Hospital
3501 Johnson Street
Hollywood 33021

Duval County Family
Planning Project
Planned Parenthood of North
East Florida
2255 Phyllis Street, Suite 101
Jacksonville 32204

Lee Davis Health Center
Hillsborough County Health
Department
2313 East 28th Avenue
Tampa 33605

GEORGIA

Grady Memorial Hospital
Emory University Family
Planning Program
Family Planning Service
68 Butler Street
Atlanta 30319

Richmond County Health
Department
Family Planning Project
Augusta 30902

*Kennestone Hospital
Church Street
Marietta 30060

Burke County Health
Department
Waynesboro 30830

HAWAII

Hawaii Planned Parenthood
200 North Vineyard
Boulevard
Honolulu 96817

IDAHO

Lewis-Clark Family Planning
Services
North Central District
Health Department
Lewiston 83501

ILLINOIS

Northwest Suburban
Vasectomy Clinic
1430 North Arlington
Heights Road
Arlington Heights 60004

*McNeal Memorial Hospital
3249 South Oak Park
   Avenue
Berwyn 60402

Cook County Hospital
Fantus Out-Patient
   Vasectomy Clinic
1825 West Harrison Street
Chicago 60612

*Illinois Central Hospital
5800 Stony Island Avenue
Chicago 60637

Illinois Masonic Medical
   Center
836 West Wellington Avenue
Chicago 60657

*Michael Reese Hospital and
   Medical Center
2929 South Ellis Avenue
Chicago 60616

Midwest Population Center
100 East Ohio Street
Chicago 60611

Planned Parenthood of
   Chicago
185 North Wabash Avenue
Chicago 60601

*Presbyterian–St. Luke's
   Hospital
1753 West Congress Parkway
Chicago 60612

*University of Illinois Hospital
Box 6998
Chicago 60612

*Sherman Hospital
Center Street
Elgin 60120

People's Health Center
215 East Stephenson Street
Freeport 61032

INDIANA

Marion County General
   Hospital
960 Locke Street
Indianapolis 46202

*Methodist Hospital of
   Indiana
1604 North Capitol Avenue
Indianapolis 46202

Planned Parenthood of North
   Central Indiana
Memorial Hospital Vas
   Clinic
615 North Michigan Street
South Bend 46601

Planned Parenthood of Vigo
   County
1024 South 6th Street
Terre Haute 47807

IOWA

*Sartori Memorial Hospital
6th and College
Cedar Falls 50613

*St. Luke's Methodist
   Hospital
1026 A Avenue, N.E.
Cedar Rapids 52402

*University of Iowa Hospitals
   and Clinics
Newton Road
Iowa City 52240

*Allen Memorial Hospital
1825 Logan Avenue
Waterloo 50703

*Schoitz Memorial Hospital
Ridgeway and Kimball
    Avenues
Waterloo 50702

KENTUCKY

Northern Kentucky Family
    Planning Project
Division of Maternal and
    Child Health
315 East 15th Street
Covington 41011

*Ephraim McDowell Hospital
217 South Third Street
Danville 40422

*Harlan Appalachian Regional
    Hospital
Martins Fork Road, Box 960
Harlan 40831

University of Kentucky
    Medical Center
800 Rose Street
Lexington 40506
(Contact: Planned
    Parenthood of Lexington
331 West Second Street
Lexington 40507)

*Jewish Hospital
217 East Chestnut Street
Louisville 40202

*Methodist Hospital
315 East Broadway
Louisville 40202

LOUISIANA

*Ochsner Foundation Hospital
1516 Jefferson Highway
New Orleans 70121

MAINE

Maine Medical Center
22 Bramhall Street
Portland 04102

MARYLAND

Johns Hopkins Hospital
601 North Broadway
Baltimore 21205

*Maryland General Hospital
827 Linden Avenue
Baltimore 21201

Peoples Free Medical Clinic
3028 Greenmount Avenue
Baltimore 21218

Planned Parenthood
    Association of Maryland
517 North Charles Street
Baltimore 21201

*Sinai Hospital, Inc.
Belvedere Avenue at Green
    Spring
Baltimore 21215

Cooperative Vasectomy
    Clinic
Prince George's County
    Planned Parenthood
6737 George Palmer
    Highway
Seat Pleasant 20027

140 *THE TRUTH ABOUT VASECTOMY*

MASSACHUSETTS

*Beth Israel Hospital
330 Brookline Avenue
Boston 02215

*Cambridge Hospital
1493 Cambridge Street
Cambridge 02139

Boston Family Planning
 Project Vasectomy Service
79 Paris Street
East Boston 02128

Lemuel Shattuck Hospital
170 Morton Street
Jamaica Plain 02130

*Marlboro Hospital
57 Union Street
Marlboro 01752

*Waltham Hospital
Hope Avenue
Waltham 02154

*Memorial Hospital
119 Belmont Street
Worcester 01605

MICHIGAN

The Washtenaw County
 League for Planned
 Parenthood
313 North First Street
Ann Arbor 48103

Planned Parenthood of South
 West Michigan Vasectomy
 Clinic
997 Agard Street
Benton Harbor 49022

Planned Parenthood League,
 Inc.
Professional Plaza Concourse
 Building
3750 Woodward Avenue
Detroit 48201

Riverside Clinic
8445 East Jefferson Avenue
Detroit 48214

*General Hospital
30712 Michigan Avenue
Eloise 48132

Planned Parenthood
 Association of Kent
 County
425 Cherry S.E.
Grand Rapids 49502

Population Council, P.C.
26111 Woodward
Huntington Woods 48070

*Foote Memorial Hospital
East Street
Jackson

*Edward W. Sparrow Hospital
1215 East Michigan Avenue
Lansing 48912

Tri-County Family Planning
 Clinic
Medical Center West
 Building, Suite 405
701 North Logan Street
Lansing 48915

West Michigan Shore Line
 Family Planning Program
Muskegon County Health
 Department
Muskegon 49440

*Pontiac General Hospital
Seminole at West Huron
Street
Pontiac 48053

*Oakland Center Hospital
120 West Eleven Mile Road
Box 309
Royal Oak 48068

*South Haven Community
Hospital
South Bailey Avenue
South Haven 49090

MINNESOTA

*Glenwood Hills Hospital
3901 Golden Valley Road
Golden Valley 55422

*Fairview Hospital
2312 South Sixth Street
Minneapolis 55406

*Hennepin County General
Hospital
Fifth and Portland
Minneapolis 55415

University of Minnesota
Hospitals
412 Union Street, S.E.
Minneapolis 55455

St. Paul–Ramsey Hospital
and Medical Center
University at Jackson Street
St. Paul 55102

MISSISSIPPI

University of Mississippi
Medical Center
2500 North State Street
Jackson 39216

MISSOURI

*University of Missouri
Medical Center
807 Stadium Road
Columbia 65201

*Menorah Medical Center
4949 Rockhill Road
Kansas City 64110

Planned Parenthood
Association of Greater
Kansas City
4950 Cherry Street
Kansas City 64113

*St. Louis County Hospital
601 South Brentwood
Boulevard
St. Louis 63105

*St. Luke's Hospital
5535 Delmar Boulevard
St. Louis 63112

Washington University
School of Medicine
Wohl Hospital Building,
Barnes Hospital Complex
4960 Audubon Avenue
St. Louis 63110

MONTANA

Planned Parenthood of
Missoula County
Room 213, Health
Department, Courthouse
Annex
Missoula 59801

NEBRASKA

Family Planning Center
3830 Adams
Lincoln 68504

University Hospital
University of Nebraska
42nd Street and Dewey
  Avenue
Omaha 48105

NEVADA

*Sunrise Hospital
3186 Maryland Parkway
Las Vegas 89109

District Health Department
  Clark County
625 Shadow Lane
P.O. Box 4426
Las Vegas 89106

Planned Parenthood of
  Washoe County
Medical Arts Building
505 North Arlington
Reno 89502

NEW HAMPSHIRE

Hitchcock Clinic
2 Maynard Street
Hanover 03755

NEW JERSEY

*Atlantic City Hospital
1925 Pacific Avenue
Atlantic City 08401

*Cooper Hospital
6th and Stevens Streets
Camden 08103

*Cherry Hill Medical Center
Chapel Avenue and Coopers
  Landing Road
Cherry Hill 08034

Morris Area Planned
  Parenthood Vasectomy
  Clinic
19 East Blackwell Street
Dover 07801

*John F. Kennedy
  Community Hospital
James Street
Edison 08817

*Elizabeth General Hospital
  and Dispensary
925 East Jersey Street
Elizabeth 07201

New Jersey Center for
  Infertility
485 Route 9W
Englewood Cliffs 07632

Hunterdon Medical Center
Route 31
Flemington 08822

*Paul Kimball Hospital
600 River Avenue
Lakewood 08701

Monmouth Medical Center
300 Second Avenue
Long Branch 07740

*Montclair Community
  Hospital
120 Harrison Avenue
Montclair 07042

*Burlington County Memorial
  Hospital
175 Madison Avenue
Mount Holly 08060

*Jersey Shore Medical Center
  (Fitkin)
1945 Corlies Avenue
Neptune 07753

*New Jersey College of
  Medicine and Dentistry
Martland Hospital Unit
65 Bergen Street
Newark 07107

*United Hospitals Medical
  Center
15 South 9th Street
Newark 07107

*Barnert Memorial Hospital
  Center
680 Broadway
Paterson 07514

*Princeton Hospital
253 Witherspoon Street
Princeton 08540

*Salem County Memorial
  Hospital
Woodstown Road
Salem 08079

*Shore Memorial Hospital
New York and Sunny
  Avenues
Somers Point 08244

*Medical Center of Vineland
2815 East Chestnut Avenue
Vineland 08360

NEW MEXICO

*Bataan Memorial Hospital
5400 Gibson Boulevard
Albuquerque 87108

*Bernalillo County Medical
  Center
University of New Mexico
  School of Medicine
2211 Lomas Boulevard, N.E.
Albuquerque 87106

Bernalillo County Planned
  Parenthood Association,
  Inc.
113 Montclaire, S.E.
Albuquerque 87106

NEW YORK CITY

Bronx–Lebanon Hospital
  Center
1276 Fulton Avenue
Bronx 10456

Downstate Medical Center
450 Clarkson Avenue
Brooklyn 11203
Attn: Dr. Robert E. Hackett

Family Planning Resources
  Center
Sixth Floor—44 Court Street
  at Joralemon Street
Brooklyn 11201

Long Island College Hospital
340 Henry Street
Brooklyn 11201

*Maimonides Medical Center
4802 Tenth Avenue
Brooklyn 11219

*Williamsburg General
  Hospital
757 Bushwick Avenue
Brooklyn 11211

Bellevue Hospital Vasectomy
  Service
First Avenue and East 27th
  Street
New York, N.Y. 10016

Margaret Sanger Research
  Bureau Vasectomy Service
17 West 16th Street
New York, N.Y. 10011

Mount Sinai Medical Center
Fifth Avenue and 100th
  Street
New York, N.Y. 10029

New York Medical College
Flower–Fifth Avenue
  Hospital
1249 Fifth Avenue
New York, N.Y. 10029

Twenty-Second Street Center
380 Second Avenue
New York, N.Y. 10010

NEW YORK STATE

*Albany Medical Center
  Hospital
New Scotland Avenue
Albany 12208

Deaconess Hospital of
  Buffalo
1001 Humboldt Parkway
Buffalo 14208

*Millard Fillmore Hospital
3 Gates Circle
Buffalo 14209

Dobbs Ferry Medical
  Pavilion
88 Ashford Avenue
Dobbs Ferry 10522

*Nassau County Medical
  Center
2201 Hempstead Turnpike
East Meadow 11554

*Charles E. Wilson Memorial
  Hospital
33-57 Harrison Street
Johnson City 13790

*Nassau Hospital
Second Street
Mineola 11501

*Northern Westchester
  Hospital
East Main Street
Mount Kisco 10549

*DeGraff Hospital
445 Tremont Street
North Tonawanda 14120

*Genesee Hospital
224 Alexander Street
Rochester 14607

*Highland Hospital of
  Rochester
South Avenue and Bellevue
  Drive
Rochester 14620

Planned Parenthood League
  of Rochester and Monroe
  Counties
38 Windsor Street
Rochester 14605

*Rochester General Hospital
1425 Portland Avenue
Rochester 14621

*Strong Memorial Hospital of
  the University of Rochester
260 Crittenden Boulevard
Rochester 14620

Metropolitan Medical
  Associates Vasectomy
  Clinic
521 Main Street
Sparkill 10976

Planned Parenthood of
  Syracuse
1120 East Genesee Street
Syracuse 13210

*Upstate Medical Center
750 East Adams Street
Syracuse 13210

NORTH CAROLINA

*Stanly County Hospital
North 4th Street
Albermarle 28001

North Carolina Memorial
  Hospital
University of North Carolina
Chapel Hill 27514

*Duke University Medical
  Center
Durham 27706

*Watts Hospital
Club Boulevard and Broad
  Street
Durham 27705

North Carolina Baptist
  Hospital
300 South Hawthorne Road
Winston-Salem 27103

NORTH DAKOTA

*Dakota Hospital
South University Drive
Fargo 58102

*Grand Forks Clinic
Grand Forks 58201

*Good Samaritan Hospital
Williston 58801

OHIO

*Akron City Hospital
525 East Market Street
Akron 44309

Vasectomy Services, Inc.
3333 Vine Street
Cincinnati 45220

*University Hospitals of
  Cleveland
2065 Adelbert Road
Cleveland 44106

Planned Parenthood
  Vasectomy Clinic
Hattie W. Lazarus Center for
  Family Planning
206 East State Street
Columbus 43215

*Riverside Methodist Hospital
3535 Olemangy River Road
Columbus 43214

*Miami Valley Hospital
1 Wyoming Street
Dayton 45409

Planned Parenthood
  Association of Miami
  Valley
124 East Third Street
Dayton 45403

OKLAHOMA

Comanche County Family
  Planning Project
P.O. Box 5255
Lawton 73501

*Norman Municipal Hospital
901 North Porter Street
  Box 1308
Norman 73069

Planned Parenthood
  Association of Oklahoma
  City
740 Culbertson Drive
Oklahoma City 73105

Planned Parenthood
  Association of Tulsa
1615 East 12 Street
Tulsa 74120

OREGON

*Josephine General Hospital
Grants Pass 97526

*Bess Kaiser Hospital
5055 North Greely Avenue
Portland 97217

*McKenzie–Willamette
  Hospital
1460 G Street
Springfield 97477

PENNSYLVANIA

Geisinger Medical Center
Danville 17821

*Easton Hospital
21st and Lehigh Streets
Easton 18042

*General Hospital of Monroe
  County
East Brown Street
East Stroudsburg 18301

Monroe County Planned
  Parenthood Association
P.O. Box 76
East Stroudsburg 18301

*Harrisburg Hospital
South Front Street
Harrisburg 17101

*Lancaster General Hospital
555 North Duke Street
Lancaster 17604

*Albert Einstein Medical
  Center
York and Tabor Roads
Philadelphia 19141

*Episcopal Hospital
Front Street and Lehigh
  Avenue
Philadelphia 19125

*Graduate Hospital of the
  University of Pennsylvania
19th and Lombard Streets
Philadelphia 19140

*Hospital of the University of
  Pennsylvania
106 Dulles Building
3400 Spruce Street
Philadelphia 19104

*Pennsylvania Hospital
Eighth and Spruce Streets
Philadelphia 19107

Planned Parenthood
  Association of South East
  Pennsylvania
1402 Spruce Street
Philadelphia 19102

Presbyterian–University of
  Pennsylvania Medical
  Center
51 North 39th Street
Philadelphia 19104

Temple University Medical
Center
3401 North Broad Street
Philadelphia 19140

Magee–Women's Hospital
Forbes Avenue and Halket
Street
Pittsburgh 15213

*Montifiore Hospital
3459 Fifth Avenue
Pittsburgh 15213

Planned Parenthood of
Pittsburgh
526 Penn Avenue
Pittsburgh 15222

*Reading Hospital
Sixth Avenue and Spruce
Street
Reading 19602

*Guthrie Clinic Ltd.
Sayre 18840

*York Hospital
1001 South George Street
York 17405

RHODE ISLAND

Lying-In Hospital
50 Maude Street
Providence 02908

Planned Parenthood of
Rhode Island
47 Aborn Street
Providence 02903

SOUTH CAROLINA

Charleston County Health
Department
334 Calhoun Street
Charleston 29401

Medical University Hospital
80 Barre Street
Charleston 29401

TENNESSEE

*Erlanger Hospital
Wiehl Street
Chattanooga 37403

*City of Memphis Hospital
860 Madison Avenue
Memphis 38103

*Methodist Hospital
1265 Union Avenue
Memphis 38104

*Morristown Hamblen
Hospital
North High Street
Morristown 37814

TEXAS

Arlington Public Health
Center
120 West Main
Arlington 76010

Dallas Family Planning
Project
2600 Stemmons—Suite 162
Dallas 75207

Planned Parenthood of
Dallas
3620 Maple Avenue
Dallas 75219

*Providence Memorial
Hospital
1901 N. Oregon
El Paso 79902

*South El Paso Hospital
702 East Paisano
El Paso 79901

John Peter Smith Hospital
  Vas Clinic
Tarrant County Hospital
  District
1500 South Main Street
Fort Worth 76104

Ben Taub General Hospital
  Vas Clinic
Harris County Hospital
  District
1502 Taub Loop
Houston 77025

Hermann Hospital Vas Clinic
1203 Ross Sterling Avenue
Houston 77025

Planned Parenthood of
  Houston
3512 Travis Street
Houston 77002

*Bexar County Hospital
  District
4502 Medical Drive
San Antonio 78229

VERMONT

*Medical Center Hospital of
  Vermont
Colchester Avenue
Burlington 05421

Planned Parenthood of
  Vermont
16 Church Street, Room 8
Burlington 05401

VIRGINIA

University of Virginia
  Hospital
Jefferson Park Avenue
Charlottesville 22901

*Fairfax Hospital
3300 Gallows Road
Fairfax 22046

WASHINGTON

*Kadlec Methodist Hospital
1005 Goethals Street
Richland 99352

Harborview Medical Center
325 Ninth Avenue
Seattle 98104

*Northwest Hospital
1551 North 120th Street
Seattle 98133

Population Dynamics
  Vasectomy Service
3829 Aurora Avenue North
Seattle 98103

U.S. Public Health Service
  Hospital
1131 14th Avenue South
Seattle 98114

*Tacoma General Hospital
315 South K Street
Tacoma 98405

*WASHINGTON, D.C., see
  DISTRICT OF
  COLUMBIA*

WEST VIRGINIA

Memorial Hospital
3200 MacCorkle, S.E.
Charleston 25304
Attn: Dorothea Fee, R.N.

*West Virginia University
  Hospital
Morgantown 26506

WISCONSIN

*Beaumont Clinic Ltd.
1821 South Webster Avenue
Green Bay 54301

*Mt. Sinai Medical Center
948 North 12th Street
Milwaukee 52233

Planned Parenthood
  Association of Milwaukee
1135 West State Street
Milwaukee 53233

*Plymouth Clinic
1000 Eastern Avenue
Plymouth 53073

APPENDIX C
SEMEN BANKS

The two most active firms in the business of freezing human semen for later use in artificial insemination are Genetic Laboratories, Inc., and Idant Corporation.

Genetic Laboratories has offices at 2233 N. Hamline Ave., St. Paul, Minn. 55113; 342 E. 67th St., New York, N.Y. 10021; 3333 W. Peterson, Chicago, Ill. 60645; 10921 Wilshire Blvd., Los Angeles, Calif. 90024; and 450 Sutter St., San Francisco, Calif. 94108. The company plans to establish banks in other major cities.

Idant Corporation is headquartered at 645 Madison Ave., New York, N.Y. 10022, and has a branch in the Baltimore area at 23–25 Walker Ave., Pikesville, Md. 21208. Idant expects shortly to have branches operating in Boston, Chicago, Los Angeles, San Francisco, Detroit, Denver, Dallas, and Portland, Ore. Long-range plans include Idant banks in Atlanta, Miami, San Diego, St. Louis, Tokyo, and London.

According to AVS, the following organizations are reported to be operating semen banks and/or research facilities:

J. K. Sherman, Ph.D.
Department of Anatomy
University of Arkansas
  Medical Center
4301 West Markham
Little Rock, Arkansas
  72201

Edward T. Tyler, M.D.
The Tyler Clinic
921 Westwood Boulevard
Los Angeles, California
  90024

Robert R. Quinlan,
  Director
Chartered International
  Cryobank
710 Bush Street
San Francisco, California
  94108

Colorado Sperm Bank
3865 Cherry Creek North
  Drive
Denver, Colorado 80209

Melvin Cohen, M.D.
Michael Reese Hospital
2929 South Ellis Avenue
Chicago, Illinois 60616

S. J. Behrman, M.D.
Department of Fertility
  and Family Planning
University of Michigan
Ann Arbor, Michigan
  48104

Emil Steinberger, M.D.
University of Texas
  Medical School
Houston, Texas 77025

Pre-Birth Clinic, Inc.
1028 Connecticut Avenue,
  N.W.
Washington, D.C. 20036

INDEX

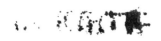